No man can reveal to you aught but that which already lies half asleep in the dawning of your knowledge.
~ Kahlil Gibran

The
PATH

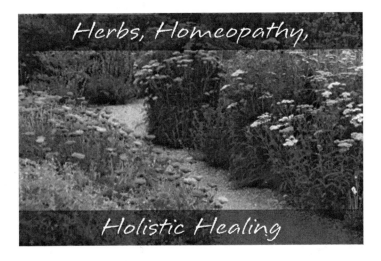

Herbs, Homeopathy,

Holistic Healing

A Resource Guide To
Everyday Wellbeing

Joyce L. Graham

The Path: Herbs, Homeopathy, Holistic Healing
by Joyce L. Graham

Published by
Graham New Vision, LLC
Joyce@JoyceGraham.com
www.JoyceGraham.com

Editing by Betsy Zelinger, www.theezeditor.com
Cover and Interior Layout by Nick Zelinger, www.nzgraphics.com

ISBN: 978-0-9858279-0-8

Library of Congress Control Number: 2012914610

First Edition 2012

Printed in the United States of America

Disclaimer:
This book is intended for educational purposes only. If you have a medical condition, seek the advice of a licensed medical practitioner.

For Thomas

CONTENTS

Introduction

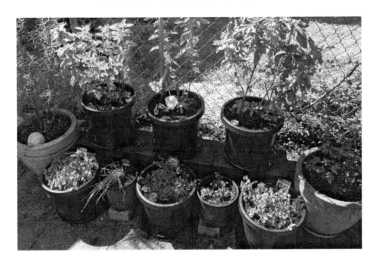

Introduction

*How many of us wonder how to determine
which herb or homeopathic remedy to use?*

*How many of us don't know how to find
a practitioner to talk to?*

It has been both a gift and a privilege in my life to serve others on their journey toward better health: physically, emotionally, and as a result, spiritually. It is my sincere intention, as the editor of this book, to introduce you to some primary herbs, basic homeopathic remedies, and holistic healing resources that will light your way toward a new path for reaching your personal goals. While in school, one of my teachers said, "Learn a few good remedies, and then you will have a great resource at your fingertips. You cannot learn them all." I've always remembered that teacher and felt that it was sage advice. To know a few effective remedies that work well for you—your being, your mind, and your spirit—will suffice in almost all cases.

The chapter on herbs in this book, written by Brigitte Mars, a well-known herbalist, is rich with healthy herbal recommendations and teas you can prepare easily. My chapter on homeopathic remedies offers helpful information that can be useful in acute situations. The third section of this book consists of essays and stories generously shared by practitioners in private practice whose knowledge, dedication, and joy enlivens their experience with clients and improves the quality of their clients' lives. I hope *The Path* will similarly help enrich your personal well-being.

To not be in a hurry is a wise practice. Use this simple and easy to comprehend book as an educational tool and deepen your understanding. Take it in your suitcase to be a guide when you travel. *Sharing is caring*, so, help your family, friends, and co-workers learn about the natural, holistic path.

Joyce L. Graham

A Few Great Herbs

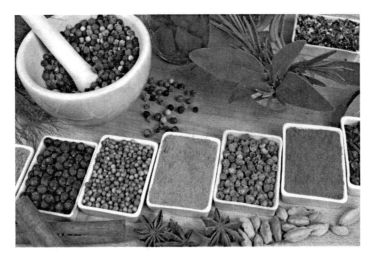

Since the beginning of life as we know it, we have been surrounded, in Mother Nature's garden, by a variety of plants, grasses, weeds, shrubs, trees, and herbs.

History shows us that plants have been used in a variety of creative ways for shelter, food, clothing, dyes, musical instruments, transportation, and medicine. Local healers, shamans, midwives, indigenous tribes, and those who synthesize medicines have used the practice of herbalism. The practice is holistic, which means that the whole person is considered in the treatment of the symptoms.

The following chapter was written by well-known herbalist Brigitte Mars to introduce *A Few Great Herbs* to you in a joyfully holistic and healthy way. Be sure to linger over the tea-making section. It's a delight to read.

A Few Great Herbs

~ Brigitte Mars ~

Thousands of plants can be known and used. However, knowing just a few of them can be very versatile and fulfill many human needs for food, tea, medicine, and many other comforts.

Catnip (*Nepeta cataria*) is a member of Lamiaceae (the mint family). It is also known as catmint, catnep, catswort, field balm, and nep.

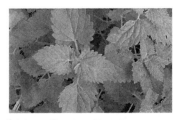

The genus name, *Nepeta*, derives from a Roman town named Nepeti where the herb was first cultivated. The common name "*catnip*" refers to the attraction cats have for this plant. Its smell has an effect similar to the pheromones that cats secrete, and it seems to affect them in a euphoric, aphrodisiacal way. Approximately two-thirds of cats will respond to catnip by sniffing, drooling, licking, rolling, stretching, rubbing, and so on.

Catnip leaf contains calcium, magnesium, chromium, B-complex vitamins, vitamin C, essential oils (cavracol, citronellol, geraniol, nepetol, nepetelactone, pulegone, thymol), iridoids, and tannins.

Energetically, catnip is considered pungent, bitter, cool, and dry. Catnip contains nepetelactone, which is both analgesic and sedative and which affects the opioid receptor sites of the body. Catnip moves chi, relaxes the nerves, and calms inflammation. This is an excellent herb for children. It will help ease them through the trials of teething, colic, and restlessness. When given for colds and fevers, it helps the patient get the rest he or she needs.

Today, catnip is used to treat amenorrhea, anxiety, bronchitis, chickenpox, colds, colic, convulsions, delayed menses, diarrhea, dyspepsia, fever, flatulence, headache, hives, hyperactivity, hysteria, indigestion, insomnia, measles, menstrual cramps, mental illness, motion sickness, pain, pneumonia, restlessness, scarlet fever, smallpox, stomachache due to nerves, teething pain, toothache, and worms.

Topically, catnip can be used in a bath to relieve stress, colic, and teething pain. A compress or poultice made from it can treat pain, sprains, bruises, hemorrhoids, or toothache. It also can be used as: a hair rinse to relieve scalp irritations and dandruff, a lotion for the treatment of acne, a liniment to alleviate arthritis or rheumatism symptoms, an enema to cleanse the colon, a salve to soothe hemorrhoids, or an eyewash to relieve inflammation, allergy symptoms, or bloodshot eyes.

The leaves can be smoked both as a euphoric and to stop hiccups. The essential oil is used in perfumery. Tying the dried herb up in an old sock makes a great catnip toy for cats. The scent repels rats and many other insects. The dried leaves can be sewn into a sachet and placed in a pillow to help induce sleep. (It isn't just attractive to domesticated cats. Lions and tigers also often have an affinity for it.)

Young catnip leaves can be made into pesto or added to other sauces or salads. The leaves can also be used as a meat rub for flavoring. Before Chinese tea became popular in the West, catnip tea was a common beverage.

Large doses of the tea can be emetic (vomit-inducing). When smoked, the herb is mildly hallucinogenic, although no toxicity has ever been reported. It is not recommended for use during pregnancy.

In the garden, catnip is best grown from seed because it tends to draw more attention from neighborhood felines when transplanted. Hence, the saying, "If you set it, cats will eat it. If you sow it, cats won't know it."

Echinacea (*Echinacea purpurea, E. angustifolia, E. pallida*) is a member of the Asteraceae (daisy family). It is also known as rudbeckia, Missouri snakeroot, 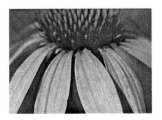 Kansas snakeroot, snakeroot, purple coneflower (E. purpurea), and Black Sampson (E. angustifolia). The name echinacea is derived from the Greek word *echinos,* which means "hedgehog," as the flowering head of this plant is stiff and bristly. The species' names are from the Latin. *Purpurea* means "purple," *angustifolia* means "narrow-leaved," and *pallida* means "pale," in reference to this plant's pale-colored petals.

The root, rhizome, leaf, flower, and seed contain beta-carotene, vitamins C and E, calcium, chromium, polysaccharaides (inulin), glycosaminoglycans, echinacoside, echinaceine, isobutylmines, caffeic acid, chicoric acid, linoleic and palmitic acids, essential oils, glycosides, polyacetylenes, sesquiterpenes, betaine, and tannin.

Energetically, echinacea is considered pungent, bitter, cooling, and dry.

Echinacea is an excellent anti-infection agent. It is most effective when taken at the onset of symptoms. The herb stimulates the formation of leukocytes and enhances phagocytosis. It inhibits the enzyme hyaluronidase, which aids the infection process by thinning cellular matrix, thereby making cells more permeable to infection. Echinacea also stimulates wound-healing and has cortisone-like activity. One of its constituents, echinacin, exhibits interferon-like activity. Another constituent, properdin, helps neutralize bacterial and viral blood toxins and increases the total number of immune cells being developed in the bone marrow. Echinacea also exhibits some antitumor activity.

In addition to its ability to ward off or mitigate illness, echinacea is used in the treatment of the following: abscess, acne, allergy, blood poisoning, boils, bronchitis, cancer, candida, chicken pox, chronic fatigue, colds, diphtheria, ear infection, eczema, fever, flu, gangrene, herpes, laryngitis,

Lyme disease, lymphatic congestion, mastitis, measles, mumps, pneumonia, prostatitis, scarlet fever, sinusitis, smallpox, snake bites, sore throat, tonsillitis, tuberculosis, typhoid, and urinary tract infections. It also can lessen the side effects of vaccinations.

Applied topically, echinacea stimulates the reticulo-epithelial layers of skin, increases the formation of antibodies, and speeds tissue repair. It is excellent when used in salves, compresses, and washes to treat cuts, boils, burns, carbuncles, gangrenous tissue, hives, infected wounds, sties, tendonitis, and venomous bites such as those from scorpions and spiders. It can be used in mouthwashes to treat canker sores, gingivitis, or pyorrhea.

Echinacea was used in Native American sweat lodges to help the participants endure the extremely high temperatures; its effectiveness can perhaps be attributed to its cooling properties. It has also been used with spiritual offerings and prayers. Echinacea has an aromatic, earthy flavor. The leaves are edible but rarely used as food, as they are prickly and have a bitter taste.

Overuse of echinacea can cause throat irritation, nausea, dizziness, and excessive salivation. Rare cases of allergic reactions have been reported. Those who have a compromised immune system, such as might result from an autoimmune illness like lupus, should use echinacea only under the advice of a qualified health-care professional. Echinacea can be taken frequently (every couple of hours) during acute infection, but this sort of dosing should only be undertaken for a few days. Herbalists disagree about the effectiveness of the herb's long-term use; many recommend taking it for cycles of ten days to three weeks, with breaks in-between, while others recommend it for continuous, long-term use. Echinacea commonly produces a slightly tingly sensation on the tongue, which is a harmless reaction.

Echinacea will grow in a wide variety of soil conditions. It prefers full sun and has low watering requirements.

Overharvesting from the wild, especially of *E. angustifolia*, is leading to endangerment of this genus. When you purchase this herb, please make sure it has been organically cultivated rather than wild-crafted.

Garlic (*Allium sativum*) is a member of the Liliaceae (lily family). It is also known as "the stinking rose." The name garlic is derived from an Anglo-Saxon 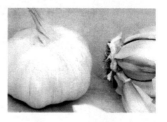 term, *leac*, meaning "pot herb" and *gar*, meaning, "lance shape," based on the shape of the leaf. The origin of the genus name *allium* is uncertain, though it is possibly linked to the ancient Greek *aglis* or Celtic *all*, meaning "burning" or "pungent." *Sativum's* species name means "cultivated."

The bulb, which is composed of cloves of garlic, contains allicin, essential oils (diallyl disulphide, diallyl trisulphide, and ajoene), sulphur, germanium, and selenium.

Energetically, garlic is considered pungent, hot, and dry. The slaves that built the pyramid of Cheops were fed rations of garlic to give them strength. Dr. Albert Schweitzer used it to treat cholera, typhoid, and typhus infections. Garlic helps protect against many types of infectious diseases, including staphylococcus, streptococcus, and salmonella bacteria. Garlic is also used to treat many circulatory system problems such as arteriosclerosis because it helps to prevent blood platelet aggregation. In addition, garlic is used to treat asthma, candida, catarrh, diabetes, high blood pressure, high cholesterol, obesity, tuberculosis, whooping cough, and worms.

Topical applications include being used as a suppository for hemorrhoids (uncut clove), bolus for yeast infections, and as an enema for dysentery. The diluted oil is used in treatment of ear infections and as a wash for gangrenous wounds and snakebites.

Eating garlic is said to repel mosquitoes, ticks, and vampires. It was worn to give protection against bubonic plague. Sailors once wore it to try to ward off being shipwrecked. Planting garlic in the garden helps repel pests.

Garlic has been a popular flavoring since ancient times and used in many parts of the world. The bulb is used to flavor meats, grains, soups, tomato dishes, salads, sauces, and breads. At garlic festivals, such as the one held in Gilroy, California, one even can taste treats such as garlic ice cream. Garlic loses its medicinal properties when heated.

Excessive use can provoke anger and emotional irritability. Bad-tempered people should avoid it. An excess amount can be irritating to the stomach and kidneys. It can also cause excessive sexual arousal, (which might be a reason to include more of it!). Note that some people are allergic to garlic.

"Garlic breath" can be a problem, as the herb remains in the body for up to ten hours. It can be overcome by chewing a mixture of anise, caraway, cumin or fennel seeds, pieces of cinnamon and parsley, or by drinking a cup of water with one drop of pure peppermint oil in it.

Do not apply cut garlic directly to the skin for more than a few minutes. It can burn the skin, so dilute the garlic with vegetable oil. Avoid large doses of it during pregnancy and while nursing as it may cause digestive distress to both mother and baby.

Garlic is believed to be native to Central Asia. It is a perennial found growing in damp pastures, woodlands, and, of course, in gardens.

Ginger (*Zingiber officinale*) is a member of the Zingiberaceae (ginger family). The origin of the name ginger is from the Indic languages of Asia, and the word means "shaped like a horn."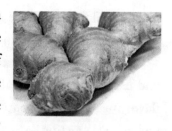

Ginger's rhizome contains sulfur, protein, proteolytic enzyme (zingibain), bisabolene, oleoresins, starch, essential oils (zingiberene, zingiberole, gingerols, shogoal, camphene, cineol, borneol, and citral), acetic acid, and mucilage.

Energetically, ginger is considered pungent, sweet, bitter, warm, and dry.

Ginger has been found to be more effective than Dramamine in curbing motion sickness, without causing drowsiness. As a digestive aid, it warms the digestive organs, stimulates digestive secretions, increases the amylase concentration in saliva, and facilitates the digestion of starches and fatty foods. It also strengthens the tissues of the heart, activates the immune system, prevents blood platelet aggregation and leukotriene formation, and inhibits prostaglandin production, thus reducing inflammation and pain. Ginger is often included in other herbal formulas, especially those that contain laxative herbs to reduce gripe.

The dried root is hotter than the fresh one and is more effective in relieving nausea and warming the body. Fresh ginger is considered the best to use for respiratory problems, but dried ginger is better for digestive ailments.

Ginger root is used in the treatment of amenorrhea, angina, ankylosing spondylitis, anxiety, arthritis, asthma, atherosclerosis, bloating, bronchitis, cancer, catarrh, chemotherapy side effects, chills, intermittent claudication, colds, colic, cough (with white phlegm), cramps, delayed menses, depression, dyspepsia, erectile dysfunction, fatigue, flatulence, flu, food poisoning, gastritis, headache, high cholesterol, hypertension, hypothyroidism, indigestion, irritable bowel, laryngitis, low libido, lumbago, menstrual cramps, migraines, morning sickness, nausea, obesity, pain, poor circulation, post-anesthesia nausea, Raynaud's disease, low sperm count and motility, stomach ache, vertigo, wheezing, and worms. It is also used to prevent blood clots, strokes, and heart attacks.

Topically, ginger can be prepared as a compress and applied over: arthritic joints, bunions, sore muscles, and toothaches to relieve pain, the kidneys to relieve the pain and assist in the passage of stones, the chest or back to relieve asthma symptoms, or the temples to relieve headaches. Ginger is wonderful when used in a bath for cases of chills, muscle soreness, sciatica, and poor circulation. It can be used in foot soaks to treat athlete's foot or to relieve the head congestion associated with colds and flu. It also can be brewed as a tea and gargled to relieve a sore throat.

In folk magic, ginger is included in spells to attract love, prosperity, and success.

Ginger leaves can also be used as a flavoring agent. Ginger root adds a pungent warming quality to soups, vegetables, Asian and Jamaican dishes, desserts, sauces, and beverages such as chai, beer, and soda. Slices of pickled ginger are often served with sushi. Candied ginger is a popular snack that helps calm nausea. Ginger powder is sometimes added to curry powders and Ethiopian spice blends and is an ingredient in five-spice powder. Brewed ginger makes an aromatic tea with a pleasant, zesty bite. The flowers can also be made into a tea with a similarly spicy but milder flavor.

Although ginger can relieve morning sickness, pregnant women should not ingest more than 1 gram daily. Avoid ginger in cases of peptic ulcers, hyperacidity, or other hot, inflammatory conditions. Avoid excessive amounts of ginger in cases of acne, eczema, or herpes. Ginger may cause adverse reactions when used in combination with anticoagulant drugs such as Coumadin or aspirin. If you are using medications such as these, seek the advice of a qualified health-care practitioner before using ginger.

The ginger plant thrives when planted in a partially shaded area with fertile, moist, well-drained soils. For gardens in temperate climates, the plant needs to be brought indoors when the cold weather begins.

Ginkgo (*Ginkgo biloba*) is a member of the Ginkgoaceae (ginkgo family) and is known by other names such as "Buddha's fingernails," the grandfather and 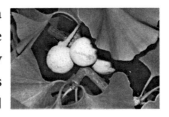 grandson tree, the maidenhair tree, and the fossil tree. The word ginkgo is derived form the Chinese word ginkyo that means, "silver apricot." The species name *biloba* is from the Latin *bis* meaning "double" and *loba* meaning "lobes," in reference to its two-lobed leaves.

Ginkgo leaf is harvested when it's starting to turn yellow and then dried. It contains beta-carotene, vitamin C, super-oxide dismutase, flavonoids (ginkgolide, quercetin, rutin, kaempferol), ginkgolic acid, terpene lactones ginkgolides, bilobalide, bilobetin, ginkgolides, and proanthocyanidins.

Energetically, ginkgo is considered sweet, bitter, neutral, and dry.

Ginkgo is the one of the oldest tree species on the planet. It was present when dinosaurs roamed the earth. It has a high resistance to disease, insects, and pollution.

Ginkgo leaf helps relax blood vessels, improving circulation and the delivery of nutrients—including oxygen and glucose—throughout the body, including the brain. It strengthens fragile capillaries and interferes with platelet-activating factor, which is a protein that can trigger spasms in the lungs. Concentrated ginkgo leaf increases the synthesis of dopamine, norepinephrine, and other neurotransmitters. Ginkgo leaf is used in the treatment of allergies, altitude sickness, Alzheimer's disease, angina, anxiety, arteriosclerosis, asthma, prevention and treatment of blood clots, bronchitis, cataracts, cough, dementia, depression, dizziness, dysentery, eczema, erectile dysfunction, fatigue, hearing loss, hemorrhoids, high cholesterol, leg cramps, leucorrhoea, macular degeneration, memory loss, nerve-related deafness, optic neuropathy, pain in the extremities, poor circulation, Raynaud's disease, senility, shortness of breath, tinnitus, tuberculosis, varicose veins, vertigo, and vision loss. It is also used to prevent and/or speed recovery from strokes.

Ginkgo leaves can be placed inside books to prevent bugs and worms from eating the books. The inner seeds are edible if boiled or roasted. The leaves are not generally consumed as a food.

Side effects from using ginkgo leaves are rare. However, large amounts have been reported to cause gastrointestinal disturbance, irritability, restlessness, and headache.

Ginkgo leaf can negatively affect the blood's ability to clot, so avoid ginkgo for at least a week before surgery, or in cases of hemophilia, or in concurrence with anticoagulant drugs such as Coumadin, aspirin, or monoamine oxidase inhibitors.

Fruit from the female trees may cause contact dermatitis or mouth lesions. Do not eat the pulp of the fruit. (It smells like dog poop, so who would want to?) Even standing over seeds while they are being roasted can cause eye irritation and dermatitis.

Mints (*Mentha* spp., especially *M. x piperita* (peppermint) and M. spicata (syn. *M. viridis;* spearmint) are members of the Lamiaceae (mint family).

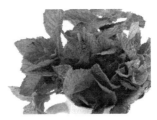

In mythology, Minthe, a Greek nymph, was one of Pluto's lovers. His jealous wife, Persephone, turned Minthe into a peppermint plant. *Piperita* is from the Latin and translates to "like pepper," in reference to its peppery taste. The species name *spicata* means "like a spire" in reference to the terminal spikes of its flowers.

The aboveground plant contains Beta-carotene, B-complex vitamins, vitamin C, potassium, flavonoids (luteolin and rutin), essential oils (menthol, menthene, methyl acetate, limonene, cineol, and pulegone), ketone (menthone), tannins, and resin. Menthol is more predominant in peppermint, and carvone is more predominant in spearmint.

Energetically, mint is considered pungent, sweet, dry, cool (at first), and warm (subsequently).

Mint relaxes the peripheral blood vessels, calms smooth muscle spasms, dries dampness, expels phlegm, and clears the head. It is considered an excellent remedy for stomach cramps, due to its ability to reduce hypercontractility of the intestinal muscles. It is often added to formulas containing laxative herbs, such as cascara sagrada, to prevent intestinal gripe.

Peppermint is considered the strongest mint, medicinally, though the other mints have medicinal benefits as well. Peppermint is effective for a wide range of pathogens, including streptococcus, staphylococcus, and candida. Spearmint is a better choice for culinary endeavors and is slightly less cooling than peppermint.

Mint is used for the treatment of colds, colic, cough, diverticulitis, dizziness, dyspepsia, earache, emphysema, fainting, fatigue, fever, flatulence, flu, gallstones, halitosis, headache, heart palpitations, herpes, hiccups, hives, indigestion, irritable bowel, laryngitis, lung inflammation, measles, menstrual cramps, morning sickness, nausea, rash, sinusitis, sore throat, stomachache, and vomiting.

Topically, mint is analgesic and anesthetic. Warm compresses of mint can be used to treat back pain, joint inflammation, lung infection, neuralgia, rheumatism, and sinusitis, while cold compresses can be used to treat bruises, fever, headache, and hives. Mint can be used as a bath herb to cool and refresh the body and to treat bug bites, chicken pox, itchy skin, and measles. The herb can also be prepared in a steam inhalation to treat asthma, bronchitis, laryngitis, nausea, shock, and sinus congestion. In a mouthwash, mint can freshen the breath and prevent gingivitis. Essential oil of mint is added to massage oils used for chest congestion and pain. Its essential oil is inhaled for asthma, bronchitis, sinus congestion, shock, and nausea, and it's also used to flavor and create antibacterial toothpastes: mouthwashes that can freshen breath and prevent gingivitis. Essential oil of mint is also used to scent soaps and shampoos and to repel mosquitoes and scabies. Ancient Athenians rubbed mint leaves on their arms to bolster their endurance. Mint was once used as a strewing herb on dirt floors. It was also stuffed into mattresses to discourage bed bugs and other vermin. Peppermint is used to clear negative energy by burning it as incense, rubbing it on furniture, strewing it in a room, or using it as potpourri.

In folklore, it is used for purification, attracting love, promoting healing, and enhancing psychic abilities. Sanitary engineers sometimes use peppermint oil to test for leakage in pipes: following its odor can locate leaks. Adding peppermint oil to a paste prevents mold and increases its shelf life. Mint essential oil is used to make mentholated tobacco products. The smell of mint repels rats and mice and has long been used to keep them out of grain storage buildings. Mint attracts bees and butterflies to a garden, and when planted near cabbages and tomatoes, helps keep them pest-free.

Spearmint is a better choice for culinary arts. It is slightly less cooling and medicinal-tasting. Mint leaves are edible raw or cooked and are often used in Middle Eastern and Asian cuisine. Use fresh leaves as a liner for cake pans.

Add either type of mint to yogurt dishes, fruit salad, vegetable salad, hummus, sauces, split-pea soup, or tabouli salad. Add mint tea to dilute fruit juices or lemonade or to make ice cubes. Mint ice creams, jellies, sauces, candies, gums, and liqueurs are popular worldwide. Mint combines well with chocolate. Mint improves the flavor of other medicines and is included in syrups and lozenges as a flavoring and a medicine in its own right. Use peppermint or spearmint to make refreshing, cooling, summer-iced teas, sun teas, or cold-water infusions. Mint is often used to improve the flavor of other teas or to prevent intestinal gripe when using laxative herbs such as senna.

Mint has a familiar, flavorful, fresh taste. It is often used to improve the flavor of other teas. Spearmint has a milder flavor than peppermint. Pregnant women should ingest no more than 1 to 2 cups of peppermint tea daily. Nursing mothers should avoid large amounts of mint, which can dry up breast milk.

Mints thrive in partial shade to full sun. They like moderate to high amounts of water and are not particular about what kind of soil they will grow in. They are perennials and tend to grow in colonies. Plant mint in your garden where you don't mind it spreading, as it has a tendency to take over. And if mint is threatening the rest of your garden, put handfuls of it to good use.

Nettles (*Urtica dioica, U. urens*) are members of the Urticaceae (nettle family). They are also known as stinging nettle, common nettle, big sting nettle, 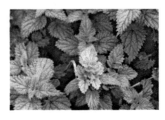 ettle, devil's leaf, devil's plaything, hokey-pokey, hidgy-pidgy, Indian spinach, ortiga, seven-minute-itch, tanging nettle, and true nettle.

The word nettles is possibly derived from the Anglo-Saxon word *noedl,* which means needle. It may refer either to the use of nettles as a textile fiber or to their sharp prickles. Other sources believe the word nettles comes from the Latin *nassa,* meaning net, as their strong stems were once woven into fishing nets. The genus name *urtica* is from the Latin meaning, "I burn." The species name *dioica* means "two dwellings" or "two houses," in reference to nettles having either male or female flowers on respective stems of different plants.

The aboveground plant contains protein, beta-carotene, xanthophylls, vitamin B, vitamin C, vitamin E, vitamin K, flavonoids (quercetin, rutin, kaempferol, and rhamnetin), calcium, chromium, iron, silica, betaine, mucilage, tannin, chromium, silica, chlorophyll, albuminoids, agglutinin, amines (histamine, acetylcholine, serotonin, and 5-hydroxy aliphatic acid), hydroxycoumarins, mucilage, saponins (lignin, and sitosterol), glycosides, and tannin.

Energetically, nettles are considered salty, slightly bitter, cool, and dry.

This herb improves just about everything! My friend David Hoffmann, author of *The Holistic Herbal*, says, "When in doubt, use nettles."

Nettle usage increases the body's resistance to pollens, molds, and environmental pollutants. It stabilizes mast cell walls, which stops the cycle of mucous membrane hyperactivity, and it nourishes and tones the veins, improves the veins' elasticity, reduces inflammation, and helps prevent blood clots. It also helps by curbing the appetite, cleansing toxins from the body, and energizing, which makes it a motivating ally for those who want to stay on a healthy diet. Drinking nettle tea before and after surgery helps build the blood, promotes healthy blood clotting, speeds recovery, and helps the patient reclaim his or her energy.

Nettle is used in the treatment of acne, amenorrhea (due to blood or kidney deficiency), anemia, arthritis, asthma, atherosclerosis, boils, bronchitis, candida, catarrh, cellulite, cystitis, diabetes, dysentery, eczema, edema, food allergies, hay fever, headache, hemorrhage, hemorrhoids, hives, hypoglycemia, infertility (men and women), jaundice, kidney stones, leukemia, lumbago, menorrhagia, mononucleosis, nephritis, night sweats, obesity, pleurisy, postpartum hemorrhage, premature gray hair, psoriasis, rheumatism, rickets, sciatica, sinusitis, tuberculosis, varicose veins, and vitiligo. It is also an excellent herb to take to speed up convalescence.

The nettle plant's individual parts have some targeted uses. Nettle leaf and root, in particular, are taken to tone and firm tissues, muscles, arteries, and skin. Taken internally, they decrease uric acid buildup and increase circulation to the skin's surface. The leaf can be used to prevent hair loss, while the root is used in the treatment of prostatitis.

Nettle seed both detoxifies and improves the ability of the liver and kidneys to cleanse the blood. Because of this, it is an antidote to poisonous plants and is useful in cases of spider bites, bee stings, dog bites, and snakebites. It is also used in the treatment of erectile dysfunction, goiter, and hypothyroidism, and it can be used to prevent hair loss.

Nettle is very stimulating when used for a process known as "urtication" that dates back at least 2,000 years. Urtication is extremely quick acting. It produces a rush of blood to the body's contacted area, which causes a counter-irritation that reduces inflammation and gives temporary pain relief. Urtication stimulates energy to the nerves, muscles, capillaries, and lymphatic system. Some say nettles relieve pain partially because the nettle pain itself draws attention away from the original, deeper pain. In any case, nettle sting causes the body to secrete its own natural anti-histamines. It can help relieve the pain of arthritis, cold feet, gout, lumbago, muscular weakness, multiple sclerosis, neuritis, palsy, rheumatism, sciatica, and chronic tendonitis. In South America, nettle urtication has even been used to treat gangrene and threatened amputations.

Topically, nettle can be used as: a hair rinse to treat dandruff and hair loss, a cleanser for oily skin, a sitz bath for hemorrhoids, a wash for sunburn, a douche for vaginitis, and an enema for detoxification. Compresses prepared with nettle tea can be used to treat arthritic joints, burns, chilblains, eczema, gout, heat rash, insect bites, mastitis, neuralgia, rash, sciatica, tendonitis, varicose veins, and wounds.

Nettles have been used to make paper, rope, fiber, fabric, and even a dark green dye for coloring fabric.

In folklore, a pot of nettles placed beneath a sickbed will hasten a patient's recovery. In *The Wild Swans* story by Hans Christian Anderson (1805-1875), a princess whose eleven brothers had been turned into swans by a spell broke it by weaving each one of them a cloak made of nettles.

Nettle has many uses in the garden. When used to water plants in the garden, nettle tea stimulates their growth and makes them more resistant to bugs. Plants growing close to nettles have more potent volatile oils levels. And when added to a compost pile, nettle hastens the breakdown of organic materials.

Nettles can be described as a "superfood." They are extremely nutritive. In seventeenth-century England, the ability to make at least seven nettle dishes was one of the factors that qualified someone as a good cook.

Nettles surpass spinach in nutritional content and can be substituted for any recipe using cooked spinach. They can also be used as a substitute for beet greens, chard, or turnip greens. Cooking the nettles deactivates their sting. Another method to rid them of their sting is to puree the nettles, and use them in pesto. Drying and powdering the herb also eliminates the sting. The dried leaves can be sprinkled on salads, soups, and vegetables for their mineral-rich, salty flavor. Ducks, goats, horses, cows, and other animals that eat dried nettles experience many health benefits from them such as shinier coats and more milk and egg production.

My favorite thing to do with nettles is to make fresh nettle juice. Nettle beer or wine is a favorite of many home brew aficionados. Flavoring nettles with a bit of lemon juice or apple cider vinegar improves mineral assimilation. Nettle juice can be used to replace the animal by-product, rennet, to curdle cheese and thereby make a vegetarian-friendly cheese.

When dried nettles are placed among stored winter fruits, the fruits stay preserved longer, are more resistant to mold, and maintain their flavor better. Nettle leaves can also be wrapped around apples, pears, root vegetables, and moist cheeses to deter pests and aid in their preservation. Nettle tea has a rich, pleasant, mineral-like flavor.

All fifty species of the genus *Urtica* can be used medicinally, but I advise you to stick with the *urens* and *dioica* species unless you consult with local herbal authorities on the safety of local varieties.

Nettle is known as "stinging nettle" for a reason; avoid touching or eating the fresh plant unless it is very young and/or you are very brave. Touching the fresh plant can cause a burning rash. Wearing gloves while collecting helps prevent this, but the hairs in large plants might pierce through them. A nettle sting can be soothed with a poultice of yellow dock, plantain, or even the juice of the nettle plant itself (but good luck on obtaining this without getting more stings). However, you can learn to love the sting. I admit to collecting nettles barehanded with just a pair of scissors and a paper bag. The arthritis I was developing twenty years ago has now become a thing of the past—and I attribute its disappearance to my nettle stings.

Eating raw nettles that are not pureed or dried can cause digestive disturbances, mouth and lip irritation, and urinary problems. But these side effects are rare if the plant is pureed before ingestion and are practically nonexistent when the plant is dried.

When used appropriately, nettle can be safely used for an extended period. Only the above-ground portions of young plants should be used as food, because older plants can be irritating to the kidneys and cause digestive disturbances.

Nettles grow just about everywhere, from waste areas and roadsides to gardens, grasslands, and moist woods. In a garden, nettle spreads widely and quickly. A kind lady from Germany gave me a single plant, and now I have at least a thousand of them. Nettle can adapt to light conditions ranging from full sun to full shade, loves soil that is high in organic matter, and enjoys moderate to high watering.

Rosemary (*Rosmarinus officinalis*) is a member of the Lamiaceae (mint family).

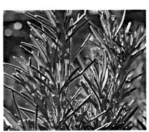

The genus and common name is perhaps derived from the Latin ros marinus, meaning "dew of the sea," as the plant grows profusely near the Mediterranean Sea coast and sea foam sprays upon it. Some etymologists think that it could have come from the Greek *rhops*, meaning "shrub," and *myron*, meaning "balm."

Rosemary is also known by the names Sea Dew and Our Lady's Rose. During the sixteenth century, Europeans carried pouches of rosemary to ward off the plague. The branches were strewn about in legal courts to prevent the spread of typhus.

Rosemary leaves tonify the nervous system, improve peripheral circulation, promote warmth, invigorate the lungs, curb infection, promote immunity, and uplift the spirits. Because it improves digestion, circulation, and memory, rosemary is an excellent herb for the elderly to take. It is used in the treatment of Alzheimer's disease, amenorrhea, anxiety, asthma, bronchitis, cataracts, cellulite, colds, debility, delayed menses, depression, dyspepsia, epilepsy, fatigue, flatulence, gallstones, halitosis, headache, hypertension, hypotension, jaundice, memory loss, menstrual cramps, migraine, pain, palsy, poor circulation, poor vision, rheumatism, stress, and vertigo.

Topically, rosemary can be used as a rejuvenating skin wash to prevent wrinkles and strengthen the capillaries, or be applied as a compress for bruises, eczema, sprains, and rheumatism. In the bath or footbath, it rejuvenates the body and mind and helps to relieve pain and sore muscles. As a gargle, it can be used to treat sore throat, gum ailments, canker sores, and to freshen the breath. Stimulating eyewashes for tired eyes can be made from it. Used in shampoos and hair rinses, rosemary deters dandruff, graying, and hair loss.

The young shoots, leaves, and flowers of rosemary are all edible, either raw or cooked. Rosemary leaves are added to vegetables, soups, breads, and jellies and used to flavor tofu, eggs, seafood, and meat dishes. Cooking with rosemary aids the digesting of fats and starches. It is included in the popular culinary blend, *Herbes de Provence*, and is used to flavor vinegars and olive oils. Rosemary has been found to be an effective food preservative that compares to BHA (butylated hydroxyanisole) and BHT (butylated hydroxytoluene).

Rosemary makes an aromatic, refreshing, pleasant, somewhat bitter-pungent piney tea. The tea is good either hot or iced. It can also be added to lemonades. Try adding a bit of ginger in to make an excellent digestive tea.

Growing rosemary provides bees with an early-season pollen plant. Rosemary has long been considered a symbol of friendship and loyalty. "Rosemary is for remembrance," is a popular, ancient saying. Ancient Greek scholars wore laurel wreaths made of rosemary on their heads to help them when taking examinations. Brides wore a wreath of rosemary and carried it in their bridal bouquets so they would remember both the families they might be leaving and their marriage vows. Rosemary was used at funerals and religious ceremonies for protection from evil and remembering the dead. It was often buried along with the dead.

Its antiseptic aroma helps prevent the spread of infection, repels many kinds of insects, and is one of the most ancient ingredients in incenses or sachets. It has been burned in sick rooms and placed inside books to deter moths. Healers wash their hands with a tea made of rosemary, because of its purifying properties, before doing healing work. Some think the herb attracts elves.

Its essential oil is widely used in massage oils, as a bath herb, and as a room spray. (Just taking ten deep inhalations of rosemary oil periodically is helping me get this chapter written.)

A yellow-green dye can be made from its flowers and leaves.

Constituents of rosemary include beta-carotene, vitamin C, calcium, iron, magnesium, phosphorus, potassium, zinc, essential oils (borneol, camphor, cineole, eucalyptol, linalol, pinene, thymol, and verbenol), tannins, flavonoids (apigenin, diosmin, heterosides, and luteolin), rosmarinic acid, rosmaricine, triterpene (ursolic acid and oleanic acid), and resin.

Rosemary is considered pungent, bitter, warm, and dry. Avoid therapeutic doses during pregnancy (although moderate use in food is all right). Though rosemary is generally considered so safe that it is a commonly used kitchen herb, extremely large doses could cause convulsions and death.

This tender perennial grows best in full sun. It needs low to moderate amounts of water, can tolerate drought if necessary, and thrives in well-drained soil.

Cayenne Pepper (*Capsicum frutescens, C. annuum, C. species*) is a member of the Solanaceae (nightshade family). Cayenne is also 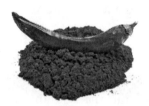 known as red pepper, African pepper, bird pepper, and chili. The genus name capsicum comes from the Greek *kapto*, meaning, "to bite," in reference to its spicy flavor. The species name *frutescens* is from the Latin *frutescere*, meaning "to fruit," or "to sprout." The common name, cayenne, refers to a town in French Guiana on the northeast coast of South America with the same name.

The fruits, also known as pods, contain beta-carotene, vitamins C and K, manganese, and capsaicin and are considered hot, pungent, and dry.

Cayenne causes more endorphin secretion in the brain, improves circulation by preventing blood platelet aggregation, and opens congested nasal passages.

Cayenne helps relieve pain, not only because of its endorphin enhancing properties, but because when it is used in diluted form, topically, it helps to block the transmission substance P, which is a neurotransmitter that transports pain messages to the brain. Cayenne is used to treat arthritis, asthma, atherosclerosis, bleeding, chills, high cholesterol, colds, coughs, dysentery, flu, migraines, and obesity.

Cayenne can be incorporated into a gargle for a sore throat. It is very effective when applied topically to bleeding wounds to stop the blood. Cayenne lotions and creams can be purchased that contain the active ingredient, capsaicin, which is applied topically to arthritic joints, sprains, shingles, and bruises. Putting a bit of cayenne between your shoes and socks on a cold winter's day helps to keep the feet warm.

Keep cayenne away from your eyes. Wash your hands after contact with any loose form of cayenne. If you ingest cayenne and it is scorching your mouth, instead of drinking water, drink milk or beer; whichever is closest, to better quell the fire. Avoid large doses when pregnant or nursing. The seeds can be especially hot and are best avoided in some varieties. Cayenne is not advised for people who sweat profusely and suddenly.

Cayenne is native to Central America. It enjoys full sun and can tolerate dry conditions.

Dandelion (*Taraxacum officinale*) is a member of the Asteraceae (daisy family). Among its many folk names are bitterwort, blowball, 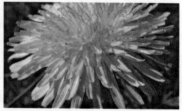 cankerwort, chicoria, clock flower, consuelda, devil's milkpail, doonhead clock, fairy clock, fortune-teller, heart-fever grass, Irish daisy, lion's tooth, milk gowan, milk witch, monk's head, peasant's cloak, puffball, priest's crown, sun-in-the-grass, swine's snout, tell time, tramp with the golden head, piddly bed, yellow gowan, wet-a-bed, and wild endive.

Opinions differ on the origin of dandelion's genus name, *Taraxacum*. Some believe that it derives from the Persian *talkh chakok*, which means, "bitter herb." Others propose that it derives from the Greek *taraxos*, "disorder," and *akos*, "remedy." Still others believe it could be derived from the Greek *taraxia*, "eye disorder," and akeomai, "to cure," as the plant was traditionally used as an eye remedy. The common name, dandelion, comes from the French *dent de lion*, which translates to "tooth of the lion," in reference to the jagged shape of the leaves.

All parts of the plant are used, but especially the leaf and root. The leaf contains beta-carotene, vitamins B1 and B2, choline, inositol, folic acid, vitamin C, calcium, iron, manganese, phosphorus, and potassium. The root contains calcium, iron, phosphorus, zinc, choline, flavonoids (lutein, luteolin flavoxanthin, and violaxanthin), pectin, and inulin.

Energetically, dandelion is considered bitter and cool.

Dandelion is one of the planet's most famous and useful "weeds." This wonderful plant is a blood purifier that aids in the process of filtering and straining wastes from the bloodstream. Dandelion cools heat and clears infection in the body. It is especially useful in treating obstructions of the gallbladder, liver, pancreas, and spleen. Dandelion is also used to help clear the body of old emotions, such as anger and fear, which can be stored in the liver and kidneys. Pregnant women will find it useful in preventing edema and hypertension.

The root is used primarily for problems related to the liver, spleen, stomach, and kidneys. Dandelion root is used to treat abscesses, acne, age spots, alcoholism, allergies, anorexia, appetite loss, arthritis, boils, breast cancer, breast tenderness, bronchitis, candida, chickenpox, cirrhosis, colitis, congestive heart failure, constipation, cysts, depression, diabetes, dizziness, dyspepsia, eczema, endometriosis, fatigue, flatulence, gallstones, gout, hangover, hay fever, headache, heartburn, hemorrhoids, hepatitis, herpes, high cholesterol, hypertension, hypochondria, hypoglycemia, jaundice, kidney stones, mastitis, measles, mononucleosis, morning sickness, mumps, obesity, osteoarthritis, ovarian cysts, poison oak and ivy, premenstrual syndrome, prostatitis, psoriasis, rashes, rheumatism, sinusitis, spleen enlargement, tonsillitis, tuberculosis, tumors, ulcers, uterine fibroids, varicose veins, and venereal warts.

The leaf, which aids in the elimination of uric acid, is used primarily for liver, kidney, and bladder concerns. The leaves help the body eliminate uric acid. Dandelion leaves are used to treat amenorrhea, anemia, anorexia, appetite loss, arthritis, bedwetting, breast cancer, breast tenderness, bronchitis, candida, colitis, congestive heart failure, cysts, debility, diabetes, dropsy, dyspepsia, edema, endometriosis, fatigue, flatulence, gallstones, hangovers, high cholesterol, hypertension, hypochondria, insomnia, kidney stones, mastitis, mononucleosis, muscular rheumatism, nervousness, obesity, poison oak and ivy, prostatitis, rashes, rheumatism, scrofula, scurvy, sinusitis, spleen enlargement, stomachache, tonsillitis, ulcers, urinary tract infection, and uterine fibroids.

Dandelion is considered one of the five most nutritious vegetables on Earth. The young leaves, gathered before the flower stalk achieves full height and the flowers have formed, may be eaten raw, used as a potherb, or juiced. The young flowers, with the green sepals removed, have a sweet, honey-like flavor and can be eaten raw. The root can be cleaned and prepared as carrots are or can be pickled. The roots are sometimes roasted and used as a coffee substitute. Dandelion wine and beer are most enjoyable.

Dandelion is generally regarded as safe, even in large amounts and even during pregnancy. However, as is true for any plant, there is always the possibility of an allergic reaction. Dandelion is a native of Eurasia but is now established in many regions around the world. Here is a free plant that can help with so many of humanity's needs! Celebrate and be grateful.

Herb tea offers an opportunity during busy days for time-outs and reflection. Rather than swallowing a couple of tasteless capsules taken with a gulp of water before running out the door, herbal tea offers time for intention. "I'm nourishing my nervous system." Or perhaps, "I'm strengthening my immune system."

Teas that are available in tea bags provide convenience for the go-go lifestyle. But herbs need to be very finely ground up before they can be put into tea bags. This grinding exposes the surface area of the herbs thousands of times, causing flavorful and therapeutic essential oils to evaporate more quickly. This is especially true when the herbs sit on a shelf for many months before being used. Many companies compensate for this by adding flavoring to the herbs.

Herbs available in loose bulk form provide better choices. Bulk herbs are less expensive and offer you the opportunity to select exactly what you want.

Store dried herbs in a glass jar or non-plastic airtight container and label them. Storing herbs near light and heat (such as in windowsills and above the stove) can deteriorate the herb quality quickly. Keep teas in a cupboard where they can be protected to better conserve their flavors and therapeutic properties. Nature will provide more herbs the next year, so don't purchase more than you are likely to use in a year.

Equipment for Tea Making

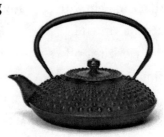

When making tea, always use fresh, cold water. Avoid aluminum cookware. Aluminum is a very soft metal and can leak a bit into the tea. The best choices for tea-making utensils are those made of glass, cast iron, stainless steel, or enamel which hasn't been chipped.

For those who can't be bothered with tea strainers, you will find tea balls or infusers in shops where herbs are sold. These perforated utensils can be filled with herbs and placed in a teapot or a pot of water for the designated amount of time. They work best when brewing leaves and flowers.

Do you need to make a lot of tea for a large group? You may want to purchase a stainless steel coffee urn and only use it to make herbal tea; otherwise, the coffee flavor will infuse your brew. Simply put the herbs in the top "basket" part, plug it in, and let it perk. This convenient method allows people to pour what they want, when they want it. This is excellent for work places, workshops, and cold weather gatherings. For health and environmental reasons, avoid Styrofoam cups. Use either washable cups or hot/cold paper cups. Wax paper cups will melt and put wax in your brew.

Tea Preparation

Use approximately one heaping teaspoon of herb tea ingredients per cup of water.

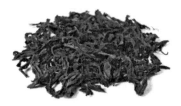

Infusion (also known as tisanes): This is an ideal method for leaves, flowers, and seeds which have delicate essential oils that would be diminished if boiled. Simply boil a cup of water and remove it from the heat. Add herb(s), cover, and allow it to steep for ten to twenty minutes. Strain the herbs into a cup before serving.

Teapot method: Fill a china or porcelain pot with hot water and allow it to stand for a minute or so. This warms the pot so the tea you pour into it will not cool down quickly, because a cold pot will impede the steeping process. Pour off the water, add loose herbs, (1 heaping teaspoon for each cup plus one extra one "for the pot"), and fill the pot with boiling water. Cover and allow the herbs and water to steep for ten minutes. To serve the tea, pour each cup through a strainer.

Decoction: This is the preferred method for roots and barks, which are harder, woodier, and which require more energy to extract their precious qualities. Simmer the herbs on low heat, covered, for about twenty minutes. Then strain and serve.

Overnight Jar Method: This is an excellent process for extracting the maximum amount of medicinal potential from an herb. Add about two ounces of root or bark, or one ounce of flower or leaf, to the bottom of a clean canning jar. Cover the herbs with boiling water, and put the lid on. Allow the herbs to steep for as long as half an hour for seeds, two hours for flowers, four hours for leaves, and overnight for roots and barks. In the morning, strain the herbs out and enjoy the nutrient-rich brew.

Avoid over-steeping herbs, as some flavors can intensify and become rather more medicinal and less pleasant. The tea can be enhanced with a touch of honey or a squeeze of fresh lemon.

Try out some of these time-tested remedies for health and well-being. Get to know a few herbs well, and you will begin to see why they have been the common medicine of the people for a long time.

Brigitte Mars is a medical herbalist and nutritional consultant who has worked with Natural Medicine for over forty years. She teaches Herbal Medicine at Naropa University, Omega Institute, Boulder College of Massage Therapy, Esalen, Kripalu, and Bauman College: Holistic Nutrition and Culinary Arts. She blogs for both the Huffington Post and the Care2 social network website. She is a professional member of the American Herbalists Guild.

Brigitte is the author of many books and DVDs, including *The Country Almanac of Home Remedies, The Desktop Guide to Herbal Medicine, Beauty by Nature, Addiction-Free Naturally, The Sexual Herbal, Healing Herbal Teas,* and *Rawsome!*

Visit Brigitte's web site at *www.brigittemars.com*

References:

Mars, Brigitte, American Herbalists Guild, *Desktop Guide to Herbal Medicine.* Laguna Beach, CA: Basic Health Publications, 2007.

Mars, Brigitte, American Herbalists Guild, *Healing Herbal Teas: A Complete Guide to Making Delicious, Healthful Beverages.* Laguna Beach, CA: Basic Health Media, 2005.

Notes for *A Few Great Herbs*

Notes for *A Few Great Herbs*

Notes for *A Few Great Herbs*

Homeopathy

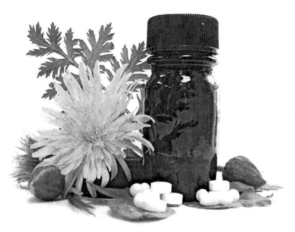

Samuel Hahnemann, a medical doctor who lived with his family and worked in Germany, founded homeopathy over two hundred years ago. This inexpensive, natural remedy for healing medical and health conditions remains remarkably popular today, in an age where patients and health care practitioners are searching for reliable, alternative solutions.

Homeopathy is a unique approach, in that it treats the signs and symptoms of the body with remedies that cause the same effects in nature. For example, Coffea Cruda, a remedy made from unroasted coffee beans, could be used to treat insomnia, excited mind, and nervousness due to overuse of coffee.

A prescription is not required, and remedies can be purchased online or in your local health food store because the ingredients are natural. Recognizing their extensive education and experience, we always recommend you work with a qualified homeopath to better serve your health needs. The homeopath considers the whole person, not just the physical symptoms, in the healing process.

The following chapter focuses on acute, short-term healing and suggests nine remedies to use to treat common ailments.

Homeopathy

~ Joyce L. Graham ~

History

Samuel Hahnemann, M.D. (1755-1843) founded the
practice of Homeopathy. He began his career and his
family in Germany. In his later years, he lived and practiced
in France. He was a medical doctor for nine years before
becoming discouraged by the current medical practices of
his day: blood-letting, purging, and using poisonous drugs.
He discovered that Chinchona bark could be used to treat
malaria symptoms. He tried this remedy on himself and
observed that when he, a healthy person, took it; it produced
the same symptoms that occurred in a person suffering from
malaria. Thus, he thought perhaps, "like cures like." Or in
other words, he thought maybe what nature provides that
causes the similar symptoms of a disease might help the
person heal from it. This idea made him interested in re-
searching and testing his theory, and it was the beginning
of homeopathy over 200 years ago.

Homeopathic remedies are made from plants, animals,
minerals, and other substances. They can be made by
repeated dilution and succussion (which means "forceful
striking on an elastic body") from the original substances,

but today they're usually made in a homeopathic pharmacy. The dosage of the remedy is determined by the amount of repeated dilutions and successions. A lower level dosage would be a 6x or a 6c. A higher dosage for a layperson would be a 30x or 30c. Most acute care remedies are in this category. When in consultation with a trained homeopath, the patient, in an acute situation, may be given a higher dosage than is readily available at the health food store.

Let me explain what we mean by "acute." These are conditions such as a cold, flu, sprain, sore back, muscle soreness, sore throat, earache, or cough. The symptoms will usually disappear if left alone, but if given the right homeopathic remedy, in the right dosage, they might have a shorter duration.

This is a most fascinating holistic practice, which, as mentioned earlier, is now over 200 years old. Most people first discover the benefit of using these remedies when they have a cold or flu, or after overeating, when they are easy to use. Athletes, bike riders, skiers, gardeners—people from all walks of life—all praise the use of one of the common remedies that helps. Most people have heard of Arnica Montana.

My intention in writing this chapter is to educate the layperson about how homeopathic remedies can be used. Further reading is encouraged to become more familiar with the field of homeopathy to understand the nature of these remedies.

Please note there are several instances when you should seek immediate medical attention. These include: high fever, bleeding, vertigo with vomiting, headaches that linger, severe vomiting, snake bites, other animal bites that are of a serious nature, or rapid heart rate.

FOR ANY CONDITION THAT IS NOT LISTED HERE, BUT WHICH SEEMS TO BE LIFE-THREAT-ENING OR OF A SEVERE NATURE, CALL 911 OR SEEK HELP FROM A MEDICAL PROFESSIONAL.

ARNICA MONTANA

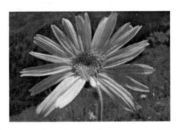

Common Names:
Leopard's Bane, Mountain Tobacco, and Sneezewort

It is quite common for a person's introduction to homeopathy to begin with Arnica. Usually after an athletic activity, a friend will recommend it, in a gel or cream form, and then it becomes a good friend to have in your home and travel-healing bag. Hikers in the Alps were allegedly the first people to use this wonderful remedy. It's easy to understand why. It's common there. They probably just broke off a sprig in the wild and, hoping it would help, rubbed some on their legs, which were screaming from the heavy climbing.

Found on the mountain sides in the USA, Europe, and Asia, it is commonly used for sprains, strains, and internal bruising. The whole plant is used when it's in flower, and it can be found formulated as a cream for external use or in homeopathic form. It is often given after a person has suffered a shock or a hard fall but does not want to go anywhere for help.

Common Uses:
- trauma
- shock from injury
- bruises, sprains, strains, contusion, after surgery, after strenuous athletic activity
- emotional shock
- concussion

General Symptoms:
- everything feels too hard
- after dental surgery or surgery of any kind
- feel as if have been "beaten"

Mental Symptoms:
- after injury or shock, patient sends his or her caregiver away and does not want help
- easily distracted
- impatient and restless
- irritable and does not want company
- seeing animals in dreams

Arnica is available in homeopathic pellets, as a cream, and in oil for massage use. The cream form should not be used on an open wound.

ARSENICUM ALBUM

Common Name:

Arsenic Trioxide

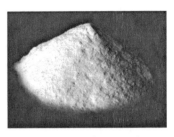

Arsenic is extracted from a mineral named arsenopyrite. It is common in its base form in Europe and Canada. In homeopathy, this remedy is highly regarded for its wide range of uses. A very small amount is used to create this remedy highly regarded for its wide range of uses.

This is a good remedy to keep with you when going out to dinner, especially while traveling. This remedy helps, if you should contract food poisoning. I gave it to a friend traveling to India, and he reported a case of food poisoning was relieved by it within a few hours after the onset of his symptoms.

Common Uses:

- anxiety, irritability, critical demeanor, panic attacks, restlessness, and trembling

General Symptoms:

- needs a lot of support from friends, family, and the doctor
- fears poverty and is an avid saver of everything
- obsessive and tries to control the environment: very fastidious
- wants to be warm; never gets too warm
- food poisoning
- is thirsty for small amounts of water

Mental Symptoms:
- anxious and worried
- very restless with tremendous anxiety
- fears being left alone and/or fears there is a burglar in the house
- perfectionist
- wants to be in control at all times
- panic attacks, especially between the hours of 12:00 to 2:00 a.m.

CHAMOMILLA

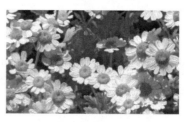

Common Names:
Corn Feverfew
and German Chamomile

The entire plant is used when preparing this homeopathic remedy. It is found growing along with corn and wheat in fields in Europe. During childhood, this is a good remedy for acute problems.

This is also a great remedy for mothers with teething babies.

Common Uses:
- helping teething babies and women after childbirth
- angry and irritable people, especially after being that way for a long time!
- generally worse before 12:00 p.m. and person feels hot
- desires to be comforted
- great for menstrual cramps

General Symptoms:
- pain seems unbearable
- angry, irritable, and complaints after anger
- teething pain
- overly-sensitive to pain
- aggravation at night

Mental Symptoms:
- irritability and anger
- infants who are irritable, especially while teething
- infant or child who can't be consoled
- abnormal sensitivity to pain
- does not want to be touched
- wants to be held and carried (children)

Symptoms Are Better:
- in warm wet weather

Symptoms Are Worse:
- anger
- heat
- cold winds in winter

COFFEA CRUDA

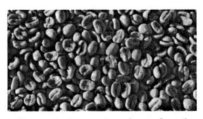

Common name:
Unroasted Coffee

Caffeine is the main ingredient. It is a stimulant for the nerves and mind and gets people up and moving in the morning. Found in Asia, Central America, and Hawaii, it is commonly grown in high-humidity mountain areas. The unroasted coffee beans are used to make the remedy.

Common Uses:
- overstimulation and excitement, strong emotions
- nervous and excited mind from too much coffee
- fatigue in overly-sensitive person
- insomnia

General Symptoms:
- insomnia with racing thoughts
- person appears thin and debilitated
- nervousness from drinking coffee

Mental Symptoms:
- racing thoughts and excited mind
- ecstatic and euphoric state
- noise and other stimuli can produce symptoms
- mild-mannered or suppressed emotions

Symptoms Are Better:
- when lying down
- when feeling warm

Symptoms Are Worse:
- overly-emotional
- cold and wintry weather

HYPERICUM PERFORATUM

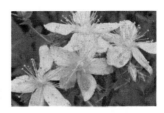

Common Names:

St. John's Wort and Woundwort

This plant has bright-yellow flowers and green leaves that ooze red juice. The secretions of its leaves are why it is called a good "blood remedy." It is a shrub and grows all over the world. The whole plant is used, while in flower, to make the remedy. It is used on areas of the body that have a large supply of nerves: fingers, toes, the spine, and the head.

Common Uses:

- treat shooting nerve pain traveling upwards
- nerve injury after an accident or after surgery
- great first-aid remedy for puncture wounds
- remedy for back pain traveling up the spine

General Symptoms:

- head injury
- found where there are many nerve endings: spine, head, fingers, and toes
- pain after childbirth in the coccyx
- falls with injury to coccyx
- pain after dental visits

Mental Symptoms:

- sleepiness
- depression

Note: this remedy may help prevent tetanus.

Symptoms Are Better:
- tilting head backward

Symptoms Are Worse:
- stuffy rooms
- damp or cold weather

LEDUM PALUSTRE

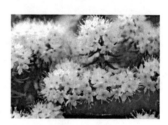

Common Names:

Wild Rosemary and Marsh Tea

This plant grows in the Northern Hemisphere: in the USA, Europe, Ireland, Scandinavia, and Canada. The whole plant is used, while in flower, and then is dried before being used to make the remedy.

This is a good remedy for rheumatic and gouty symptoms of the extremities, legs, and joints. The pain is often associated with stiffness and puffiness in the area. There is soreness, and the patient does not want to move, but will feel better after cold water bathing or using a cold compress.

Common Uses:
- puncture wounds, insect bites, and eye injuries (such as a black eye)
- rheumatic pains that travel upward in the body
- prevention of infection with wounds

General Symptoms:
- heat aggravates, symptoms lessen when cold
- helped by bathing in cold water or with ice-cold compress

Mental Symptoms:
- irritated, ill-tempered patients

Physical Symptoms:
- swelling of foot or ankle and/or desires to soak foot in cold water
- bites or stings from insects or animals
- puncture wound from a nail or sharp object
- joint pain with stiffness, feels cold

Symptoms Better:
- cold water application with compresses or cold bathing

Symptoms Are Worse:
- movement
- with heat
- wine
- in the evening

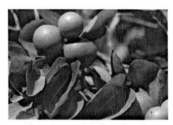

NUX VOMICA

Common Names:

Poison Nut, Quaker Buttons

This plant is a tree that grows in Australia, Burma, India, and China. The seeds contain a poison, strychnine, which is what is used to make this homeopathic remedy. It is useful for recovering from overindulgence in food, coffee, alcohol, tobacco, and overworking. People who are sensitive and highly competitive, with the "work hard; play hard ethic," may benefit from this remedy. Usually this type of person will be very impatient, overly excitable, irritable, and stubborn. They are people who like to focus on work and are very ambitious and competitive in nature.

This is a great remedy to have on hand after a holiday meal, or after overeating rich foods and/or partaking of alcohol, sweets, and coffee.

Common Uses:
- overindulgence in food, wine, smoking, coffee
- flu or colds
- overuse of stimulants or substance abuse

General Symptoms:
- fatigue from overworking
- workaholic, impatient, and irritable
- likes stimulants: coffee, wine, chocolate, and alcohol
- complains of being chilled likes being warm
- hangovers with headache

Mental Symptoms:
- anger and great irritability
- can become very angry and filled with rage
- overly sensitive to stimulation
- type A personality, very competitive
- substance abuse
- impatient
- insomnia

Physical Symptoms:
- cravings for spicy and/or fatty foods, coffee, alcohol, or any stimulant
- back pain worse at night while in bed
- cramps and sharp pains in the abdomen
- diarrhea alternating with constipation
- constipation: an urge to go, but nothing comes out

Symptoms Are Better:
- warmth
- with sleep
- in the evening
- when left alone

Symptoms Are Worse:
- cold, damp weather
- winter coldness with wind
- following stimulants or spicy foods
- mental overexertion

IGNATIA AMARA

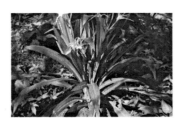

Common Name:

St. Ignatius

This plant is a small tree that is found in China and the Philippines. The remedy is made from its beans. It is similar to Nux Vomica, but has some different properties.

Often, when there has been a relationship break-up, and the patient is having a difficult time dealing with it emotionally, this is the first remedy to consider using.

Usually, it will be an unexpected shock to the patient's system. Most often, this remedy is given to women. But there are men who may need this remedy, as well.

Consider using this remedy after there's been an emotional shock: the loss of a family member, a friend's death, or any other type of grief.

Common Uses:
- emotional states: shock or hysteria, emotionally upset
- grief or loss

General Symptoms:
- laugh and cry simultaneously
- contradiction in behavior
- sensitive, artistic, sentimental, idealistic, and/or high-strung

Mental Symptoms:
- disappointment in a romantic relationship
- sensitive to being hurt
- depression

Physical Symptoms:
- headaches
- perspires only on face[a]
- lump in throat
- does not want fruit
- backache after grief

Symptoms Are Better:
- after eating
- lying on side with heat

Symptoms Are Worse:
- in the cold
- after emotional upset
- drinking coffee or smoking
- from criticism

PULSATILLA NIGRICANS

Common Names:
Pulsatilla Nigricans,
Pasque Flower,
Wind Flower

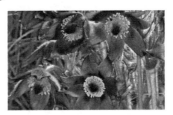

The plant grows in Europe from spring through fall and produces beautiful purple flowers. The remedy is made using the juice from the whole plant, including the flower.

Common Uses:
- green or yellow nose discharge
- digestive problems from eating fatty, rich food, nausea, vomiting
- depression
- headaches above the eye or eyes

General Symptoms:
- likes reassurance and affection
- afraid of the dark

- sensitive to changes in the weather
- eating cold ice cream causes stomach upset

Mental Symptoms:
- fears being alone
- dislikes dark places
- afraid of ghosts, insanity, and dying
- tearful for no reason

Physical Symptoms:
- aching joints
- dry mouth
- digestive complaints
- moodiness

Symptoms Are Better:
- fresh air
- receiving sympathy

Symptoms Are Worse:
- standing for long periods of time
- heat
- eating rich foods
- in the evening

Joyce L. Graham, M.S., LPC, CHom has worked in the health and wellness industry as a certified homeopath, certified Qi Gong instructor, and a licensed professional counselor for over 35 years. She is a graduate of the University of Kansas with a master's degree in psychology. She is also a graduate of the Colorado School of Classical Homeopathy and received her certification in Qi Gong from Master Lui. Her first book, *The Healer,* is a novel. She is currently working on her next book at home in Denver.

Visit her web site at *www.JoyceGraham.com* for information on her workshops and teaching schedule. She can also be contacted by e-mail. Her email address is Joyce@JoyceGraham.com.

References:

Castro, Miranda, *The Complete Homeopathy Handbook,* New York, NY, St. Martin's Press, 1990

Boericke, William, *Pocket Manuel of Homeopathic Materia Medica,* Santa Rosa, CA, Boericke and Tafel, Inc., 1927

Murphy, Robin, *Homeopathic Remedy Guide,* Blacksburg, VA, H.A.N.A. Press, 2000

Notes for *Homeopathy*

Notes for *Homeopathy*

Notes for *Homeopathy*

Every blade of grass has its Angel
that bends over it and whispers,
"Grow, grow."
~The Talmud

Holistic Healing

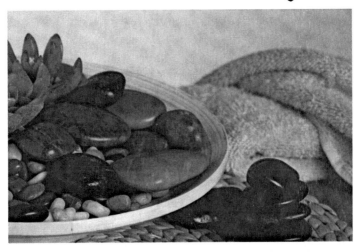

An intimate relationship with your healer / practitioner is vital to your healing process. It is one of mutual respect and is a commitment to be vulnerable and trusting. Practitioners who are guided by love and compassion lift us to a greater awareness of what is present and possible in our healing process. When this spiritual connection and conscious bond between the patient and the healer exists, a space is created where lasting changes can occur. This unity of care results in a heightened wellness for the client.

The Pillars of Chinese Medicine

~ Randel B. Wing, Lic.Ac, DOM, NMD ~

How old is Traditional Chinese Medicine (TCM)? This is a loaded question. Most of us would say thousands of years. In truth, TCM, as we know it today, began in 1965 when Mao Zedong's "Great Leap Forward" (The Cultural Revolution) was in full swing. Mao, one of world's greatest megalomaniacs, had books burned, sent all of the intellectuals to the fields (or had them killed), and brought a great many of the peasants (farmers) in to the cities to be trained to be what he called "barefoot doctors." By 1970, there were a half million of these barefoot doctors treating over a half billion Chinese people. From this, the Revolutionary Health Committee published a textbook called *A Barefoot Doctors Manual*, which was intended to equip the barefoot doctor with everything he needed to treat every condition. This book was the beginning of TCM. Today, the text is called *Chinese Acupuncture and Moxibustion*.

So, every modern student of Chinese Medicine studies Traditional Chinese Medicine (not the ancient medical practices before Mao). *Chinese Acupuncture and Moxibustion* is the main text studied to pass the national boards required for licensure. This ancient medicine is called Classical Chinese Medicine and is based upon the primary principle of Chinese Medicine, as stated in Chinese literature, which is, ***if there is free flow of Qi and Blood, there is room for nothing to go wrong*** (meaning Qi and Blood need to perform at peak performance to achieve optimum health). This flow can become blocked by negative thoughts and actions, which then cause a flood of physical and mental health problems.

The implementation has the following eight branches:

1. MEDITATION: This is considered the "great medicine." The shamans of ancient China (eight thousand years ago) believed that the world was formed from Wu Ji, which was a place of nothingness. From the Wu Ji came the Tai Qi; better known as Yin and Yang. Yin and Yang exist everywhere. One cannot exist without the other. One cannot have *up* without *down*, *black* without *white*, or *fluid* without *solid*. Yin turns to Yang. Just as the sun rises (yang energy), the sun also sets (yin energy). The Chinese say that it is highly important to spend at least fifteen minutes every day in the state of Wu Ji. This state is the one where healing takes place. How does someone reach this state? Find a place where there are no distractions. Sit or lie down and start breathing. Concentrate on the sound of your breath (in the

nose, then out the nose, with the tip of your
tongue placed at the roof of your mouth). It is
impossible to think with this type of breathing.
Try it, and you will achieve the greatest form of
medicine.

2. TAI Qi: Tai Chi Chuan/Qigong, Chinese Medicine
   in motion, emphasizes the development of internal
   energy instead of muscle strength. This internal
   energy is achieved through the feeling of one's
   breath (vital Qi) and then with the feeling of Vital
   Qi and more in-depth exercises, one develops the
   feeling of one's own internal alchemy. When the
   mind is fully centered and fully at peace, the
   possibility of changing and healing the body can
   be realized. Tai Qi is a ritual, and if practiced daily,
   can create the habit of living in the moment and
   "living in the flow."

3. NUTRITION: Food is more important than herbs
   are. Everything we feed ourselves must have good
   Qi. Nutrition not only means food, water, and air,
   it means **everything**: jobs, relationships, and what
   one sees and reads. We must always feed our souls
   with this good Qi, or the flow becomes blocked
   and health issues will develop. All foods have
   energy, except for processed foods. These foods
   are void of energy. They do not enrich our lives
   or support the "free flow." All nutritious foods

have energy. They are cold, warm, or hot. They have tastes: sweet, sour, bitter, salty, or pungent. When eating, it is necessary to do so for balance. By this, I mean if you are cold, do not eat "cold" foods (a jalapeño pepper from the freezer is still hot), but a steamed cucumber remains cold. By "balanced," I mean eating in conformance with the concepts of Yin and Yang. I refer you to the *Energetics of Food* from Meridian Press for more about this.

4. BODY WORK: This includes massage, tui na (a form of Chinese manipulative therapy), gua sha (the body surface is press-stroked with a smooth-edged instrument to intentionally raise therapeutic petechiae), yoga, pilates, and cranial sacral (the practitioner uses a very light touch at key points around the head and pelvis for this therapy). Why have this work? Because body work moves the Qi and blood, assisting and enhancing the "free flow."

5. COSMOLOGY AND PHILOSOPHY: The Chinese have always believed in **Heaven, Earth,** and **Man** (human) and the **Five Elements** (Earth, Metal, Water, Wood, and Fire). From *Heaven-Earth-Man* came the *I Ching* (or the *Book of Changes*) published by Tuttle Publishing and the concepts of *Yin and Yang*. From the Five Elements came an

understanding of the relationship of man to nature and nature to man (reference the Worsley Institute Of Classical Five-Element Acupuncture).

6. FENG SHUI: This is the Chinese system to balance geometric space by using the laws of heaven and earth to help improve the receiving of positive Qi. Feng Shui means "Wind and Water" and is associated with an understanding of nature and good health. As mentioned previously, you want everything that comes to you to have good energy or Qi. If your home or work environment is cluttered and the windows are dirty, this feeling bothers you. Remember, positive or negative feelings create "free flow" or cause stagnation. Thus, Feng Shui is about creating one's world with a sense of harmony and love.

7. HERBS: In Chinese Medicine herbs are considered food and food is considered medicine. In herbal medicine, individual herbs are seldom used separately but rather are combined using the principles of Yin and Yang and the herbs' specific functions, such as herbs that clear heat, drain damp, and cool. How did the ancients derive the use of herbs in formulations? The ancients used nature as their guideline. By this, I mean the "doctrine of signatures," which means that if a plant, animal, or mineral looked like a physical

match to something in the body, it might have medicinal value; it might be used to heal. An example of this would be the flower of the foxglove plant. The flower looks like a heart, and indeed they found this plant could be used to treat heart conditions. Today, this plant is used in modern-day medicine to produce Digitalis, which is a heart medication. For more information, I refer you to *Materia Medica* by Dan Bensky.

8. ACUPUNCTURE: Acupuncture is defined as the practice of inserting very fine needles into the body to affect the flow of Qi and Blood. Each acupuncture point along the body's energetic pathways (meridians) has a specific function, and each point has another point that is used for balance. **Balance** is always the goal and always returns to the basics of this form of medicine. *"When you have free flow, there is room for nothing to go wrong."*

Well, what do we do with this information in a clinical setting? Let's look at the following case study:

A 52-year-old female, let us call her Amy, (not her real name) presented with a chief complaint of asthma that had been diagnosed over twenty years ago. She presented with constipation, shortness of breath, poor sleep, general lethargy, and a diet that consisted of high carbs, fruits, vegetables, and dairy. Amy felt that her diet was healthy because every food item she consumed was organic. Over the years, she had been prescribed many medications, and she was ready to try another approach. She said the medications were keeping her asthma under control, but she felt unhealthy. Amy was also stressed-out because her family was paying $900 a month for health insurance, due to her medical condition. I went over a treatment plan with Amy that I thought would change her life. This plan included:

- *Acupuncture* treatments two times a week to balance the energetics of the organ systems.

- A *nutrition* diet change to eliminate phlegm production. This diet, of course, included the elimination of all phlegm-producing foods.

- Taking an *herbal* formula called Clear Phlegm.

- *Qigong* breathing instructions. This breathing involves a three-parted breath similar to yoga breathing. Once this is learned, it can become a personal way of achieving "free flow" and a source of *meditation.*

- Weekly *massage.* Amy could only afford a massage once a month, but she had a yoga tape. She could start working with that tape, and she really liked to walk. She would become more diligent about exercising.

- We talked about her personal *feng shui*, and she told me that she loved her home and garden and that she and her husband were really close to and supportive of each other.

- We also talked about what she expected. Amy wanted to achieve a sense of well-being, and I assured her this was my goal for her also.

We began treatment that day. Over the course of the next two months, Amy began to see and feel the benefits of her efforts. At the end, and in consultation with her physician, Amy was able to eliminate her asthma medications. Over the next year, she and her husband were able to clear the pre-existing diagnosis of asthma, and their health insurance was reduced to under $300 a month.

This is Chinese Medicine. Always remember to go back to basics. If you have free flow, there is nothing to go wrong.

Randel B. Wing, Lic.Ac, DOM, and NMD. Dr. Wing has a private practice in Colorado Springs, Colorado. The office name is the Premier Acupuncture Clinic. The clinic's website is *www.premieracupunctureclinic.com*. Dr. Wing has been in private practice for over fifteen years. He can also be contacted via his email address: Rwingtcmdoc@earthlink.net

References:

Twelve and Twelve in Acupuncture by Richard Tan, OMD and L.Ac., and Stephen Rush, L.Ac., San Diego, CA, 1991

The Medical I Ching; Oracle of the Healer Within by Miki Shima, Blue Poppy Press, Boulder, CO, 1992

The Practice of Chinese Medicine; The Treatment of Diseases with Acupuncture and Chinese Herbs by Giovanni Maciocia and Churchill Lingstone, New York, NY, 1994

Dao of Chinese Medicine: Understanding an Ancient Healing Art by Donald E. Kendall, Oxford Univ. Press, New York, NY, 2002

An Introduction to Aromatherapy
~ Mindy Green ~

Overview

Aromatherapy is commonly described as the therapeutic use of plant-derived, aromatic essential oils to promote physical and psychological well-being. Though the name *aromatherapy* is relatively new, the use of aromatic plants for healing, either topically or thru the sense of smell, is as old as recorded history. Every civilization with written records makes reference to the use of aromatic herbs for healing the mind, body and spirit, through ceremony in the burning of plants as incense, external use on the skin with unguents and salves, and after its discovery, through the use of extracted essential oils via distillation or cold pressing.

All herbs offer varying healing chemical components; aromatic plants have the added benefit of scent that, when used with skill and intention, can improve our mood, relax our frazzled nerves, energize our depleted bodies, and deepen our spiritual connection. Modern day practices of aromatherapy encompass topical application in skin care for cosmetic or therapeutic use and inhalation for respiratory health or mood enhancement. For the purposes of this short introduction, we will focus on the external uses for general wellness. There are hundreds of commercially available essential oils sourced from plants, but you can provide for a wide variety of uses with only a few oils. For a beginner, it is better to know a lot about a few essential oils than to know a little about many.

It is generally accepted that essential oils can penetrate the skin, enter the circulatory system, and depending upon the chemistry of the essential oils utilized, elicit varying physiological effects such as physical relaxation or stimulation, antibacterial action, supportive hormonal balancing, and more. Scent is processed in the limbic system of the brain: the same area where olfaction occurs. This is also where memory and emotions are recorded and managed. Through the sense of smell, essential oils can affect the mood, offering benefits against depression or anxiety and ease of temperament.

Safety, Dilutions, and Applications

Essential oils are highly concentrated and must be diluted for safe and effective application. The most common diluent for topical use is a "carrier" oil derived from seeds or nuts such as coconut, almond, olive, sunflower, etc.

Safety considerations:
  • Do not use essential oils undiluted

- Some citruses are photosensitizing; avoid UV light exposure for eight hours after application

- For skin and eye irritation, dilute with plain vegetable oil

- Do not use essential oils internally

Dilutions:

- Y:z % dilution = 2-3 drops of essential oil per ounce of carrier oil (for the very sensitive)

- 1% dilution = 5 drops of essential oil per ounce of carrier oil (for use on the face; for children, the elderly, or those of weak constitution)

- 2% dilution = 10 drops of essential oil per ounce of carrier oil for body massage in oil or lotion

Methods of Application:

- Massage oil with 2% dilution

- Facial Oil: Y:z to 1% dilution (in either water mist or carrier oil)

- Bath: 2-8 drops per full tub for an adult (irritants: peppermint, citrus, and spice oils)

- Foot bath: 5-10 drops per gallon of water or herb tea

- Inhalant: 5 drops essential oil in bowl of hot water with towel tent, or sprinkle on hankie

- Mists: 10 drops per one ounce water (for spraying into the air); 2 -5 drops per one ounce water (for spraying onto the skin)

Materia Medica for Ten Essential Oils

The following list is a short introduction to ten common, nontoxic essential oils with a wide range of uses. Creating blends of two to four oils will provide for a myriad of remedies, either cosmetic or therapeutic. It is best to have a good reference book for a more thorough explanation of aromatherapy and its material medica.

Boswellia carterii (frankincense) for inflammation, wound healing, skin care, or meditation aid

Citrus bergamia (bergamot) for digestive tonic, sore throat, detox, acne, lymphatic congestion, or depression: NOTE: this citrus oil is available without the photosensitizing component; look for the words "bergapten free" on the label.

Lavandula angustifolia (lavender) for insect bites/stings, sunburn, headache, bruises, sprains, acne, rash, or depression

Eucalyptus globulus (eucalyptus) for respiratory and sinus congestion, inflammation, pain, colds, flu, herpes, or shingles

Chamomilla nobile or *Anthemis nobilis* (Roman chamomile) for spasms, swelling, insomnia, or relaxation

Melaleuca alternifolia (tea tree) for athlete's foot, burns, warts, acne, cold sores, flu, or insect bites

Mentha piperita (peppermint) for indigestion, nausea, headache, fatigue, fever, sinusitis, or pain relief: substitute spearmint for pregnancy

Origanum majorana or *Majorana hortensis* (sweet marjoram) for anti-spasmodic, sore muscles, insomnia, menstrual cramps, or arthritis

Rosmarinus officinalis (rosemary) for headache, fatigue, hangover, constipation, muscle aches, or circulatory tonic

Cananga odorata (ylang-ylang) for cosmetic care for all skin types or relaxation

A Few Easy Recipes

First, a note about blending: most essential oils blend well. The key is to keep it simple. Use between two to four essential oils, and keep the total number of drops appropriate to the dilution needed for the specific application. Get creative and blend for your aromatic preference.

Relaxing Massage Oil (suitable for insomnia, stress, or depression): One ounce of coconut oil, five drops of lavender, three drops of bergamot, and two drops of chamomile

Energizing Massage Oil (suitable for mental stimulation, muscle pain, and revitalizing):
One ounce of coconut oil, five drops of rosemary, and five drops of eucalyptus

Aromatic Mists for the Environment

One of the simplest, immediately gratifying, and low-tech ways to utilize essential oils is by creating your own aromatic mists to spray into the air.

These can be used to cleanse negative energy, clear a professional office space between clients, calm yourself in traffic, energize your mood, or simply to make your home smell wonderful. In this case, the carrier diluent used is water instead of vegetable oil. These spritzers are like a fresh, cool breeze, can be used anywhere, and can be customized for almost any occasion. They are simple and safe home-made preparations that are fun to make and can be created by anyone with an adventurous spirit. These preparations may be sprayed onto the body, into the air, or on linens. Avoid misting over wood furniture with a lacquer finish. Shake well before each use; essential oils separate when added to water. The following recipes are added to one ounce of water:

Energy Clearing: five drops of frankincense, three drops of geranium, and two drops of bergamot

> *Air Purification:* (helps to reduce airborne bacteria):
> five drops of eucalyptus, three drops of bergamot,
> and two drops of tea tree

Aromatic Spritzers for the Skin

Misting the skin with these fragrant waters delivers a delightful and refreshingly cool breath of nature. The mind, body, and spirit can be rejuvenated with just a few pumps of a mist bottle filled with these fragrant offerings.

These preparations offer an added benefit in cosmetic care. The skin craves moisture to keep it youthful and supple. If you've consumed enough water to feed the skin from the inside, misting the outside of your skin is the next best thing for rehydration. Arid climates, air conditioning, dry heat, or excessive sun exposure all wreak havoc on skin, creating dehydration that contributes to fine lines. Misting the skin helps plump it up with soothing constituents from essential oils and the crucial water hydration it needs to maintain a youthful glow, no matter what type of skin you have. A fine mist will not disturb makeup and may be used several times a day, depending upon the environmental conditions.

My favorite time to mist my skin is when I'm freshly out of the shower. If you like this idea, blot your skin dry, and spray your entire body. Men can spritz their faces after shaving to help reduce shaving irritation and soothe sensitive skin. Always keep your eyes closed when misting your face. Apply a light lotion to slow the evaporation of water from the skin and seal in the moisture. Your skin will drink in the vapor, and a subtle cloud of beautiful fragrance will accompany your day.

To avoid irritation when using essential oils on the face, with water as a carrier, greater dilution is required. Mix ten drops of an essential oil blend in a two-ounce bottle (preferably glass) with a fine mist sprayer. Fill with purified water, witch hazel (for oily skin), or aloe vera juice (for dry skin). Shake well before each use, and be sure to close your eyes while spraying your face.

NOTE: Remember to avoid the use of citrus oils on skin that has been exposed to ultraviolet light (sun and tanning beds) for at least eight hours, because of possible photosensitivity and increased pigmentation.

> *Summer Cooler:* six drops of lavender, three drops of geranium, and one drop of peppermint
>
> *Lighten Up:* five drops of lavender, three drops of bergamot, and two drops of Roman chamomile
>
> *Beautiful You:* five drops of lavender, three drops of frankincense, and two drops of ylang-ylang

Why Use Essential Oils Derived from Plants?

Human beings have a biological familiarity with plants. For millions of years, we have relied on them for food, medicine, and body adornment. Our cells have come to effectively recognize and efficiently utilize the myriad of natural chemicals they provide to keep us in health and harmony with our environment. In this symbiotic relationship, our bodies have evolved with them, just as they have evolved on our planet; together we grow in ecological awareness. It is only in the last hundred years that we, as a species, have been exposed to synthetic chemicals in our medicines, foods, and cosmetics. They are often the harbingers of ecologically detrimental effects, many with proven negative or unknown consequences. The incorporation of plant ingredients demonstrates our support of a dynamic and integrated system of individual and global health.

Quality is important in true aromatherapy. Many essences are masquerading as pure essential oils, even those adulterated with synthetic ingredients. Buy your essential oils from a reputable company with a proven track record of purity. Ask your local health food store clerk to guide you, don't hesitate to call the supplier, further educate yourself, and most importantly, be sure the Latin name of the plant is on the label. I wish you many happy hours creating, inhaling, slathering, and indulging in these beautiful fragrances of nature!

Mindy Green is a co-author of the 2009 book entitled *Aromatherapy, a Complete Guide to the Healing Art.* She is an herbalist with decades of experience, an esthetician, an educator, and a lifelong student of

all things botanical. You can visit her website at
www.greenscentsations.com.

Reference Books:

Aromatherapy: A Complete Guide to the Healing Art by Kathi Keville
and Mindy Green

The Encyclopedia of Essential Oils by Julia Lawless

Essential Oil Safety: A Guide for Healthcare Professionals by Robert
Tisserand and Tony Balacs

Blazing Your Own Trail

~ Jacqueline Bambenek ~

There have been many pivotal points in my life, but the one most deeply ingrained in my heart is the one where I allowed my inner guidance to direct me to the Rocky Mountain foothills of Colorado. The Full Self Emergence Program—(I took the longest course; the eighteen-month one)—at Sunrise Ranch Spiritual Retreat Center in Loveland, Colorado, called me forward in a new direction and was the beginning of a journey in coaching, transformational classes, and living intentionally in community. When I heard the mission of their parent organization, the Emissaries of Divine Light, providing a space for the 'spiritual regeneration of humanity,' it resonated deeply with the core of my being.

My coach and I had ventured out for a relaxing walk, enjoying the brisk spring air and discussing the events that had led me to Colorado. I looked up at the beautiful backdrop of the red rimrock, feeling her strength and my connection to Mother Earth, with the gorgeous view of Green Glade Reservoir sitting majestically before me. In teachings, I had learned that water is symbolic for "the new that has yet to take form and be clarified"…which was basically everything in my life. I then noticed the 'Dead End' sign and thought how perfect it was for this discussion. I asked, "So what do you do when you are faced with this sign?" My beautiful coach looked at me and said, "Well, sweetie, you can either turn around and go back the way you came, or you can blaze your own trail."

Those words inspire me to keep my eyes focused on what I wish to create and bring into form. To make a difference—by assisting others to realize their inner potential to be magnificent creators by modeling the freedom that is offered through taking responsibility for living fully—is a passion of mine. If we chose to raise our level of awareness by doing the things that bring us joy, we would make a huge contribution toward increasing planetary consciousness.

One way that I have chosen to raise the 'joy factor' in my immediate environment is to connect with others in building community. A desire was born in me to embrace the creation and facilitation of a monthly Healers' Jamboree Sharing Circle. Many people attend because they love to experience this connection. We are blessed that Sunrise Ranch has embraced this vision with us…and is now growing to include The Glen Ivy Center in Corona, CA. My vision of this includes it becoming a regular event globally.

It is a glorious experience to share time with other practitioners in Northern Colorado and those interested in the healing arts. The tendency of the healer is to give, which is beautiful. However, all too often I have witnessed healers who rarely take the necessary time to receive and restore their energetic reserves. This was the purpose of creating the Healer's Jam: to offer support to one another and make sure we are consistently able to offer our best to our clients. We are an outlet of expression and connection among colleagues; formed to develop friendships based on honoring one another and bringing forth our special gifts, which often entails simply 'being you.'

We are at a pivotal time in history where we have a great deal to learn from one another. We are magical creators with the ability to bring our focus of thought and intention onto a positive wavelength. It is amazing to consider the positive and negative effects that words—combined with thoughts and feelings—can bring forth into our world. What an immense power we hold! When we recognize the divine nature within us that allows us to bring into manifestation that which our thoughts entertain, we have reached one of the ultimate understandings.

This amazing journey of being in Colorado has led me to climb mountains, to raft the Westwater Canyon on the Colorado River, to fall in love with the beauty of Spirit in all that is amplified in nature and all beings around me, and to accept events as they occur without judgment.

As I reflect on all of the amazing lessons that were provided on our river trip, the one that holds the greatest meaning for me is that of being one with the flow of the river. When we fight the current and paddle upstream, we get tired very quickly. There is not much distance gained in trying to fight the current. The river is energy and it is relative to our lives. When we are moving with the flow of life, we are naturally rewarded. We can enjoy the ride and live to our fullest! We are also blessed to know times of stillness, where we can get quiet within our body, mind, and spirit. When we come to a rapid, we don't want to get hung up on the boulders or on fixed points of reference. Be open to moving quickly through the rapids, often needing to steer directly into the wild, rushing river. Confront what is needed head on.

The awareness of how important *trusting my inner guidance* is and the recognition of the gift of *holding space* has been life changing for me. Welcoming the stillness and finding the radiance of love to be fully present to provide loving support has been a fun exercise in clearing the mind and appreciating the little things in my environment.

A very big step to take on this journey is facing our fears. Recently, I have found myself realizing that to move beyond the state of fear, I first needed to decide I was 'done with' self-limiting thought patterns. In order to step outside of that fear, I needed to decide what it was that I desired to step forward into. Acknowledging that we have ultimately created fears to keep us safe from pain requires a sense of gratitude. I have come to realize that I cannot live fully while staying within my comfort zone. Feeling the full expression of life does involve some risk.

One of life's greatest gifts and opportunities is trusting that life will bring us what we need to experience and work through. How far ahead of the curve we are, when we choose to allow the mind to see situations as opportunities, even during times of difficulty, as we grow in the process and learn new ways of being. We experience more expansive states of being by choosing to see the brighter side of life.

Perception can offer us beautiful insight when we open our minds to allow for greater possibility. When we choose not to limit our abilities by what our mind can conceive and begin to ask questions, instead of always seeking the answers, we allow a space for the Universe to bring forth the manifestations of our thoughts and feelings. To ask, 'What else is possible?' can create unlimited changes in our creative field.

It is my desire to encourage each of us to take responsibility for where we are, for the direction and feelings we choose to have, and how we respond to others or to ourselves. What a travesty it is to give away our power by reacting negatively to a situation. To find a point of stillness, honoring oneself, and stepping out of a situation temporarily, when needed to regain a positive point of reference, can be priceless.

In my own experience, I had to let go of many false identities. These were based on the beliefs that I was taught were important. It is amazing how quickly the house of cards can crumble around you when you don't know at the core of your being who you are. This was my experience. I had to come to the understanding that my core identity was 'love'. 'Home' is a place that resides within my heart, and I can take it wherever I go.

It is exciting to see so many people around the world wishing to live in the experience of wholeness. Focusing on building our foundational strengths of *truth, love,* and *integrity* is our key for sustainability. To offer forgiveness into the world to those who have hurt us, and to learn how to trust and love again, gives us hope for our future. When we allow the walls we have built around our hearts to dissolve, we can offer the greatest expression of ourselves into our world: love. To say, 'thank you for being the storm,' to those who have hurt us, offers us clarification of who we are and moves us in the direction we are meant to grow and learn from.

It is an amazing gift to live in community with others who wish to share in bringing their best selves forward and be in alignment with Spirit. I encourage you to honor the fact that magic can happen anywhere when you recognize the real magic comes from within your own heart.

Jacqueline Bambenek is a holistic health practitioner and energy worker. She specializes in spiritual health coaching, is a certified biofeedback technician through the Natural Therapies Certification Board, works with doTerra™ certified pure therapeutic-grade essential oils, is a certified Ersdal Zone Therapist through the Academy of Dynamic Integrative Therapy, a Reiki Master, and is certified as an Attunement Practitioner through the Attunement Guild. Jacqueline is the

Manager of Program Development for The Glen Ivy Center, which is a spiritual retreat center located in southern CA. You may reach her through her email: joy4bodymindspirit@gmail.com.

For more information, please visit the websites below:
www.vibrationalenergysolutions.com
www.glenivy.org

The Healing Process

~ Wonder Bob ~

What is Healing?

When we experience illness and disease it can be uncomfortable, unbearable, and debilitating. Many times, we assume that outside elements are creating our reality. "I picked up a virus," or "I caught a cold."

What if the idea of "catching" illness is misplaced? What if illness can only occur with imbalance in the body, energetic field, or emotional state? What then creates these states of being? Can we raise them to a higher vibration and eliminate disease?

We have learned that if our inner environment is well, the body is brilliant at healing itself. Cancers have been eliminated through change of diet or addition of supplements. Chronic disease has been relieved through the reduction of stress and body movement.

What if we have all that we need for healing? What if our bodies know how to heal themselves? Couldn't we contribute to our bodies and allow them to do what they do best?

In studying *Ascended Masters, Gurus, and Avatars,* they display a state of perfect health and awareness. They are able to heal at will, bi-locate, communicate over vast distances, manipulate matter, and generate higher states of being; even shine like a being of light. Many of these beings have declared that we will be capable of much more than they are demonstrating as human potential: "...*the works that I do shall he do also; and greater works than these shall he do (John 14:12)*. Could it be that these way-showers have been coming to us to demonstrate the potential of humans in the world?

We've heard many references to the ninety-pound mother who lifted the car off her son. She was from Lawrenceville, Georgia. She lifted a 1964 Chevy Impala off her then-teenage son. He'd jacked up and removed a rear tire and was working on the suspension. The mother found her son (Tony) caught under one of the rear wheel wells and out cold. Mom, in her late 50s, raised the car and kept it up for five minutes while neighbors pulled Tony to safety.

A thirty-five-year-old woman was trapped in her submerged SUV in a Pueblo, Colorado flood. An out-of-work store manager reached his hand inside the car and pulled her out. Other would-be rescuers couldn't break the windows, and all four windows were still closed when the SUV was towed from the river. How did this man reach through a closed window and pull this woman through the glass?

Sue (not her real name) was diagnosed with reticulum cell sarcoma, a rare bone cancer. Her body and organs had been eaten up by the cancer, and after five years of struggle and pain, she was no longer responding to treatment. The doctors informed her she was very near the end. She attended a faith healing event as a last resort. After she prayed, she experienced intense heat throughout her body. The pain disappeared and she was able to run up on the stage. Later, the doctors found no evidence of cancer.

The great teachers have been able to raise their vibrational energy, see beyond time and space, manifest food, control weather, or live off the prana (non-physical body of essential energy) of the environment. Somehow, someway, these way-showers have been able to access a higher consciousness.

Shamans in Tibet compete with each other to raise their body temperatures in extreme cold. They place wet sheets over themselves and dry them out with their chi (life force energy). What if we asked our bodies to flow chi? What could they create?

In Thailand, a man read a book about yogis who could manifest food from nothing. He then performed a prescribed meditation to create food. When he opened his hand, a grain of rice was present. How was food manifested out of nothing?

While trekking in the Himalayas, a hiker contracted a debilitating illness. As his doctors did not know what the disease was, he was treated with over-the-counter antibiotics. After much purging, he practiced pranic breathing to recover. He was well in two days. Later he discovered the illness was Legionnaire's Disease. The standard treatment time for that is several weeks. How did he heal himself in two days?

What if these people are truly able to connect to the unified field and raise their vibrations?

In these higher states, illness is just not possible. What is the key? What is the way?

The body is an obvious collection of atoms, cells, blood, muscles, organs, bones, membranes, and skin. It has an amazing intelligence, which is capable of directing movement, synapses, growth, and healing. What if we acknowledged this amazing intelligence of the body and created a dialog with it? Could we ask it how to heal itself?

A conversation to ask the body what it wants can be had. When we go grocery shopping, do we do it for us or for our bodies? If we are open to it, our body will lead us to the perfect selection of what it requires. What if we just gave it what it wanted? Wouldn't it be happier?

At the pharmacy, the body will talk to us with muscle testing and other methods. If you allow your body to lead you, it will actually pull you down the aisles that it likes. It will also register which specific products will be its best experience. What if we allowed ourselves to move toward health in this way?

We also know that something continues to exist when our body dies. Many call this the soul. Others refer to it as our energy, space, and consciousness. This awareness has existed through many cycles of reincarnation, death, and rebirth. The soul consciousness can be accessed through many methods: via meditation, hypnosis, past life regression, and reading the Akashic records. It exists as a field of energy in our bodies. Can we dialog with this field?

An easy way to access the soul consciousness is by merging with it. Expanding our awareness beyond our bodies and communities into the solar system and cosmos can do this merging. What if our soul is infinite: beyond space-time and dimensions? Is, "To infinity and beyond," truly our destiny?

Where the body and the soul intersect, the mind is created. In this reality, we operate mainly from the mind. But does the analytical, gerbil wheel of thinking keep us stuck in cycles of analysis-paralysis?

Have you ever found yourself doing a task and experienced being really pissed off? Nothing has happened that you are aware of; you're just really angry. Could it be that we run hidden mind programs without knowing it? The program may be discontinued by asking, "Is this mine?" What else can we ask ourselves?

Did you ever notice how we are addicted to the mind? Awareness and consciousness are mistranslated as "higher mind," "transcended thinking," or "mindfulness." Do we really want to be full of mind?

If we changed our language, we could transform "What do you think?" to "What do you know?" Similarly, we could change "I think that..." to "I perceive..." and being "mindful" to being "aware." What if we could create a greater awareness through our language in this way?

Physics has discovered we are holographic beings. This means that our beings contain the blueprint of the entire universe from macrocosm to microcosm. By perceiving the cosmos, couldn't we easily understand our inner being?

Operating from a see-able, touch-able world, how can we access the microcosmic zoo within our bodies? What if the planets, stars, and galaxies operate much like the cells in our bodies? If we understood the cosmos, would this awareness affect our health?

What if the simple act of observing can drastically change a physical process? In quantum physics, electrons and photons can behave as either a particle or a wave. When an observer is watching, particles are observed. When not observed, waves are present. When behaving as waves, electrons and photons can simultaneously pass through several openings in a barrier and then meet again on the other side of the barrier. This "meeting" is known as interference.

However, interference only occurs when no one is watching. As an observer begins to watch the particles going through the openings, the electrons are "forced" to behave like particles instead of waves. Thus, the mere act of observation affects the experimental findings. We know the wave potential is possible. But once the wave is observed, it becomes a particle. What if this creation phenomenon could be translated into our bodies? What a great way to bridge energy and matter.

What if everything is energy? And what if matter is simply transformed energy?

"In the beginning was the Word, and the Word was with God, and the Word was God." – John 1:1

And the Word was made flesh..." – John 1:14

What if the "Word" means "sound," "God" means "divine energy," and "Flesh" means "the physical or matter?" An expanded interpretation might be "In the beginning was the energy/sound of the divine, this vibration is part of the divine, and this vibration is divine. And this divine energy was sounded into physical being". Could it be that sound is the bridge between energy and matter? Knowing matter is simply densified energy, couldn't we work with its vibration to easily heal matter?

What if working with energy could be facilitated by connecting all the meridian points on the body? If this could open the pathways, a greater flow of chi could occur, and access to all that is would become possible. What if reclaiming these connections could shift, change, alter, or re-create any part of the body? How much healing could then occur?

Knowing that healing is possible is a huge step toward shifting any uncomfortable situation. But we get hung-up in the rightness or wrongness of the process. What if this right/wrong reality thinking prevents us from healing?

As children, we really don't care if we are right or wrong. We simply want to play in the world. We don't judge a person when we ask them, "Will you be my friend?" Only when our parents and teachers tell us to be good, do we shift our behavior into "good," according to their point of view. As we play, we might get a stern look from an adult. We then try to figure out what we are doing wrong. Then we actually make ourselves "wrong" due to someone else's judgment of our behavior!

What if being right or wrong didn't matter? What if everything was just a point of view? If significance and judgment are the wet blankets of consciousness, can we throw them off?

One of the dichotomies of this reality that we perpetrate upon ourselves is connection and significance. They are warring opposites in the human desire of fulfillment. The need for connection is achieved through relationships, friendships, romance, family, and community. Yet we have this burning desire to be significant, to be different, separate, and noticeable outside the group. If it just didn't matter, could we let it all go? Could we live our lives without being triggered: no buttons to push, and no energetic cattle prods?

A female friend felt powerless in her marriage. Because her husband was the breadwinner, her authority was often deferred to his. She developed a problematic lower back. When she went in for x-rays and treatment, she received a lot of compassion and attention. Suddenly, her back condition gave her a lot more authority over her life than what she had been getting at home. The back condition then became hugely significant. How invested in the disease was she?

Many times, we create disease and illness in our bodies in reaction to our relationships. A female client was in the hospital dying of ovarian cancer. I asked her, "What are you dying to get out of?" She gasped and then replied, "I just can't be with my husband anymore." After releasing the guilt of wanting a divorce from her field, she was able to choose divorce instead of death. The cancer went into remission after the divorce. She was defending her choice of marriage to the death, literally!

Knowing that our bodies and awareness are brilliant, couldn't we contribute to them to facilitate great change? Have you ever travelled to a new state or country and noticed how good it feels? Could it be that we can recover lost parts of our being?

A normal speed of dying allows the soul to properly detach from the body. What happens in a sudden-death scenario when the soul doesn't have enough time and space to transition? Do we leave soul fragments behind? What if the loss of fragments hinders our recovery from illness? What could be created by retrieving these soul fragments?

Entities? Really?

I never gave much credence to discarnates or non-corporeal beings. It's good to know that with a body, we are much more powerful than anything without a body. But we do allow entities and implants to play in our bodies. Most of the reception of them occurs when we are not in control of our faculties.

If we drink or take drugs, the cerebral cortex of the brain opens up like a welcome mat and says, "Come on in and play." Discarnates, implants, explants, and entities then jump into parts of our bodies and have a party of their own.

Many times the attachment creates illness or stress in the body. Removing the entity clears the energy and allows the body to shift into a greater state of health. What if this removal is a lot easier that we imagine?

Near-death experiences and past-life regressions have allowed us to look into previous incarnations. The trauma incurred from being hurt, killed, tortured, wounded, or abused may create a trauma receptor in the energetic field. From the point of creation of the traumatic event, illness is created in a specific area. What if the trauma receptor creates a reoccurring probability of illness around the injury location? What if this trauma receptor is carried through many lifetimes?

As an example, one of my clients discovered she was strangled in a past life as a roman soldier. The trauma created by the death scenario produced throat cancer, breathing disorders, and speech impediments for her in many lifetimes, including her current one. Regressing her back to the specific point of trauma allowed the memory to be rewritten. Like a stack of dominoes falling forward, the release of trauma allows the soul history to be rewritten.

Are our Light Bodies our ultimate state of healing and being?

"As Jeshua demonstrated his light being to Peter James and John on the mount of transfiguration. And after six days Jesus taketh Peter, James, and John his brother, and bringeth them up into an high mountain apart, And was transfigured before them: and his face did shine as the sun, and his raiment was white as the light. And, behold, there appeared unto them Moses and Elias talking with him."
–Matthew 17:1

"...when Moses came down from mount Sinai with the two tables of testimony in Moses' hand, when he came down from the mount, that Moses wist not that the skin of his face shone while he talked with him."
–Exodus 34:29.

"And when Aaron and all the children of Israel saw Moses, behold, the skin of his face shone; and they were afraid to come nigh him."
–Exodus 34:30.

A "light body" is described as a complete union of our aspects. A vertical pathway might be to bring our spirit and physical body into unity, becoming light. A horizontal pathway might be to bring our masculine and feminine aspects into enlightened androgyny. What if we could easily integrate these vertical and horizontal pathways? What kind of body could we create then?

What if we were able to acknowledge the intelligence of our body? What if we could ask questions like these, "Body, what kind of food would you like today? What activity would you like to participate in? Do you want to sleep now? What can I contribute to you that would allow this disease to go away?" How powerful could this conversation be?

Is BE-ing the ultimate state of health?

As an incarnate being, only you can BE you. We didn't show up to be a human DO-ing or to be someone else. And BE-ing is the key to becoming, and thus to being healthy and happy. What would you be willing to become? Ask yourself this question and ponder it for a while: try on this grand possibility.

Wonder Bob has been fascinated with personal development, healing, and awareness since childhood. He has developed a healing technique that incorporates hypnosis, shamanic tools, reiki, akashic records, energy activations, and intuitive abilities into a potent personal session. He facilitates transformative retreats, channeled information, enlightened concerts, classes on consciousness, and life-changing ceremonies.

Bob's training includes; Access Consciousness Facilitator (CFMW), Master Hypnotist (Integrated School of Hypnotherapy), Crystal Therapy, Akashic Records, Tantra (Certified Sexual Healer/Teacher), Cosmic Masters, Thai Massage, Diksha (Humanity in Unity Ashram).

Contact him via his email account:
wonder_bob@msn.com

For more information, please visit
www.conscious-heart.org

Notes for *Holistic Healing*

Notes for *Holistic Healing*

Notes for *Holistic Healing*

Listen. Make a way for yourself inside yourself. Stop looking in the other way of looking.

~ Rumi

Acknowledgments

A special thank you and much gratitude for my friends Judy Maselli and Linda Crowell who helped with reading and making changes at the last minute.

For Carolyn Peterson, Sue Tanquay, Debra Montagna, and Matt Michaels who believe in my projects and always offer their kind heartfelt support. I am so blessed to have you in my life.

To Nick Zelinger and Betsy Zelinger who work so thoughtfully and well on my designing and editing, I am honored to have your guidance and expert advice. Thank you both.

About the Author

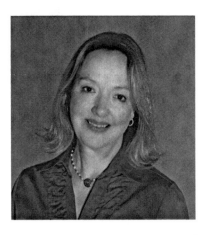

Joyce L. Graham, M.S., LPC, CHom graduated with a degree in psychology from the University of Kansas. She studied the work of Carl Jung with the inter-regional society and also at the Jung Institute in Zurich, Switzerland.

She is a licensed professional counselor, a certified classical homeopath, and a certified Qi Gong instructor. She lives in Denver, Colorado. *The Path: Herbs, Homeopathy and Holistic Healing* is her second book. Her first book, a novel, is *The Healer*.

Write to her at Joyce@Joycegraham.com and visit her web site for workshops and upcoming events at www.JoyceGraham.com.

NOW ON AMAZON

Joyce Graham's debut novel, *The Healer*
is now available on Amazon.
Visit www.Amazon.com to purchase your copy.

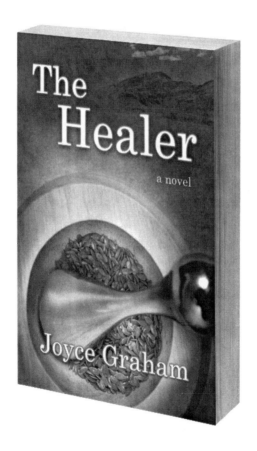

CPSIA information can be obtained at www.ICGtesting.com
Printed in the USA
LVOW131933191012

303700LV00001B/8/P